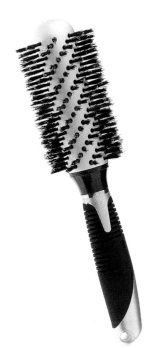

Good
HAIR

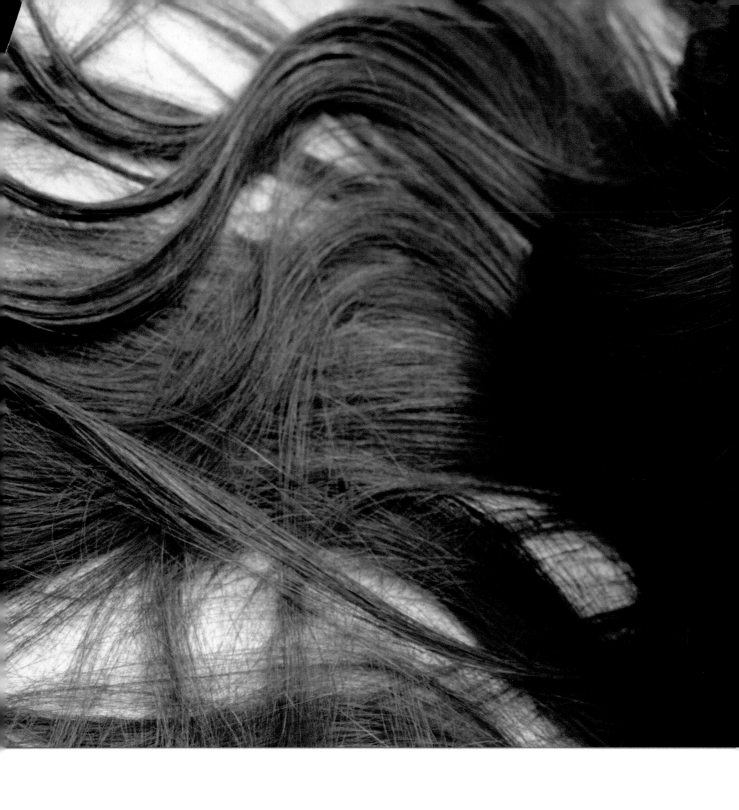

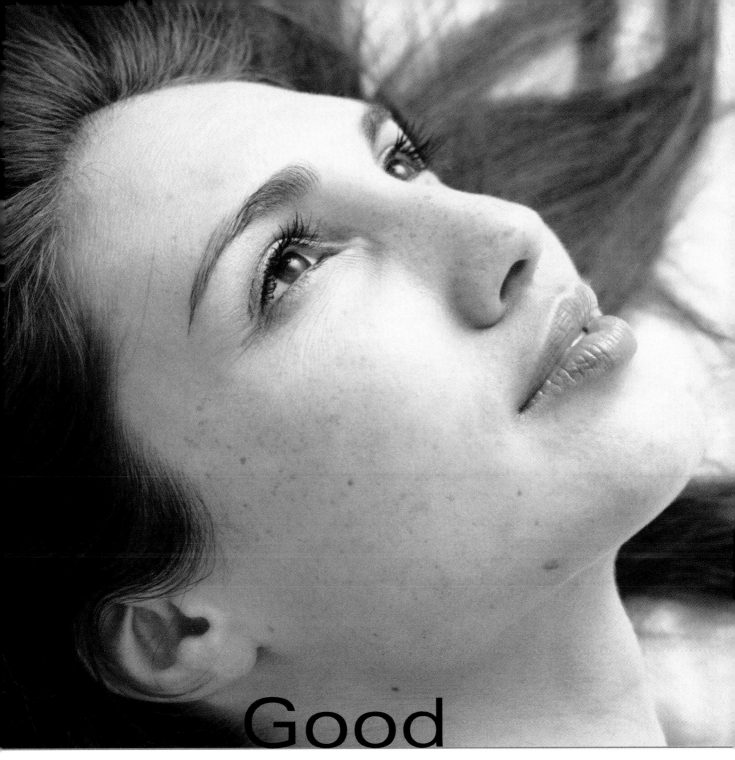

Good
HAIR

LIBBY PEACOCK

Published by Silverdale Books
an imprint of Bookmart Ltd 2006

Bookmart Ltd
Blaby Road
Wigston
Leicester
LE18 4SE

Registered Number 2372865

First published in 2005 by
New Holland Publishers
London • Cape Town • Sydney • Auckland
www.newhollandpublishers.com

Publisher: Mariëlle Renssen
Publishing managers: Claudia Dos Santos, Simon Pooley
Commissioning editor: Alfred LeMaitre
Studio manager: Richard MacArthur
Editor: Katja Splettstoesser
Designer: Elmari Kuyler
Illustrator: James Berrangé
Proofreader: Leizel Brown
Picture researchers: Karla Kik, Tamlyn McGeean
Production: Myrna Collins
Consultant: Beryl Barnard FSBTh. M.PHYS. ATT, Education
    Director, The London School of Beauty and Make-up

ISBN 1 84509 239 2 (PB)

Reproduction by Hirt & Carter (Cape) Pty Ltd
Printed and bound in Malaysia by Times Offset (M) Sdn. Bhd.

10 9 8 7 6 5 4 3 2 1

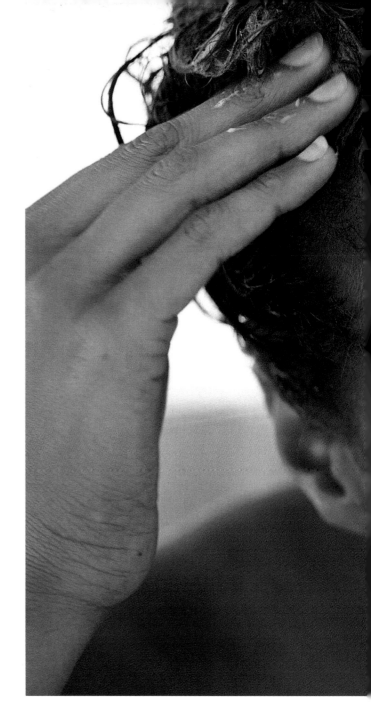

DEDICATION

This book is dedicated to all my wonderful friends. Thank you for help
me through the bad hair days!

DISCLAIMER

The author and publishers have made every effort to ensure that
information contained in this book was accurate at the time of going
press, and accept no responsibility for any injury or inconvenience sustai
by any person using this book or following the advice provided herein.

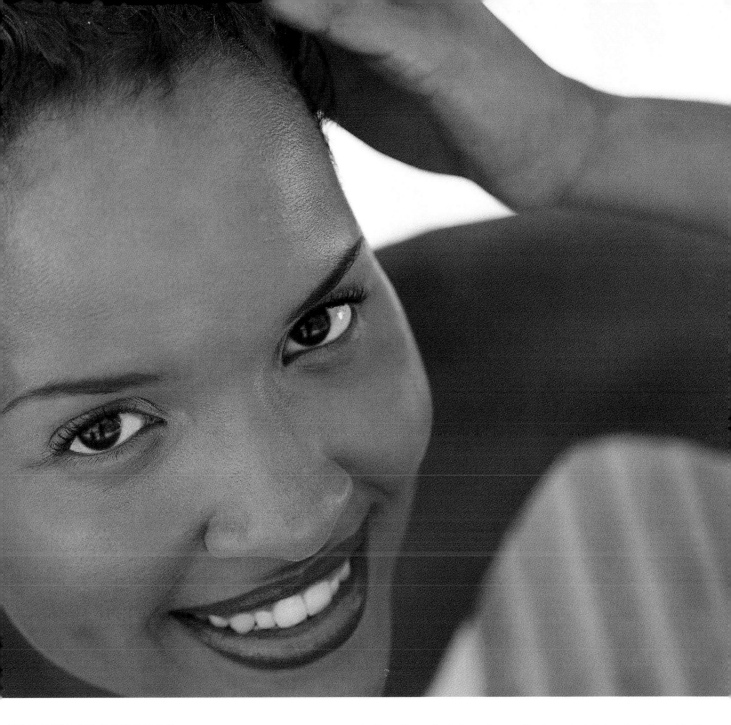

ACKNOWLEDGEMENTS

With special thanks to: Dr Sue Jessop (senior specialist and lecturer, Division of Dermatology, Groote Schuur Hospital and University of Cape Town), for advising on and checking the medical sections in *Good Hair*. Dr Larry Gershowitz and the Medical Hair Restoration Clinic in Cape Town for up-to-date information on hair transplants. Dermatologist Dr Ian Webster for information on hair-removal methods and the pros and cons of laser hair removal in particular. Julia Lovely, dietician in private practice in Cape Town, for information on the impact of diet on hair. Tony Martin of Yazo4Hair salon, for parting with expert tips on hairstyling for men and women, and for top colouring advice. Dima Tsobanopulos of D&D Designers for Hair for styling tips, and information on face shapes and the latest straightening techniques. Carlton Skincare Centre, Constantia, Cape. Skincare therapist Gerda van Rooyen for the latest on hair removal and Ellen Nwenesongole of Procter & Gamble SA (Pty) Ltd, for reference material on hair and hair products.

contents

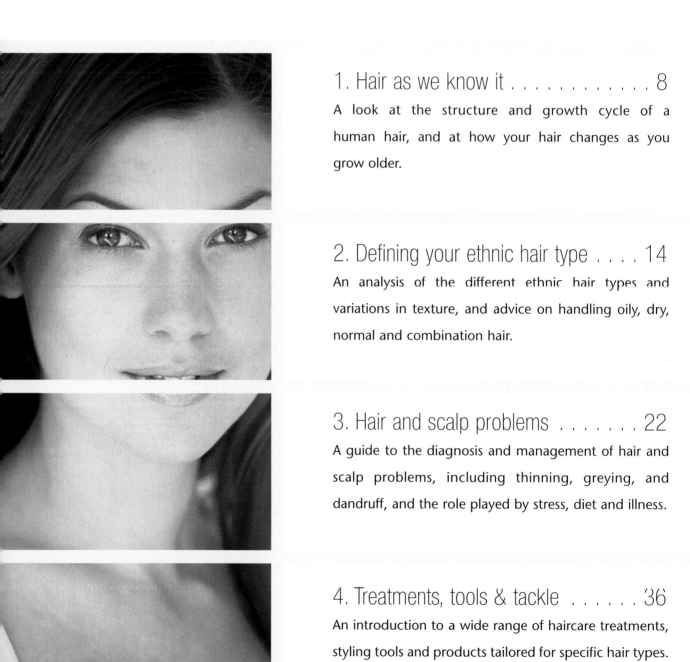

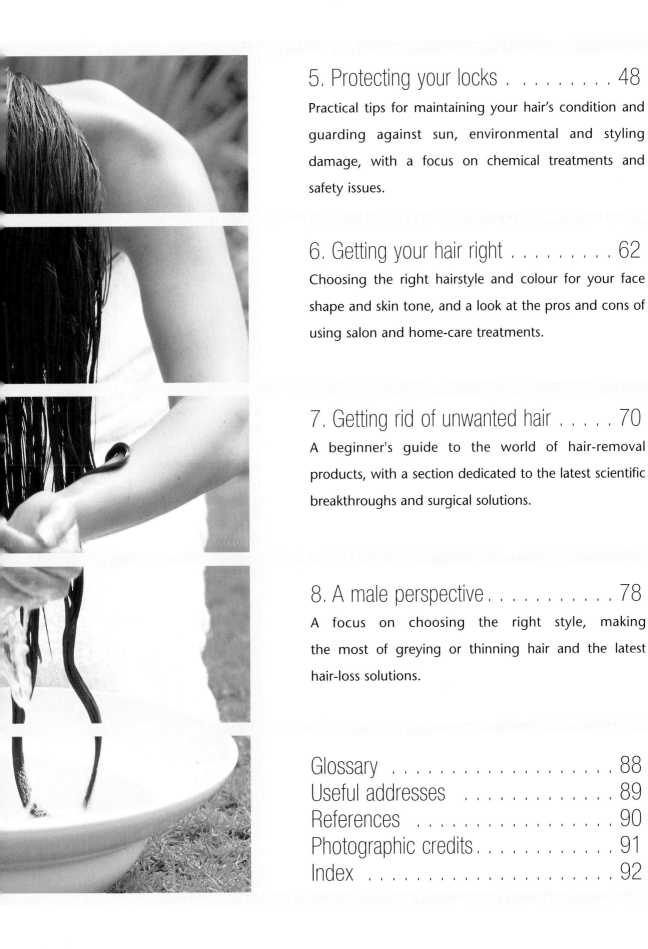

Hair as we know it

The English language is rich in hair-related expressions, for good reason: our hair is not only useful, it also reflects who we are. So, when we nitpick about small things, we split hairs; when we have a narrow escape, we escape by a hair's breadth; and when we have a good time, we let our hair down.

Hair gives away clues about our personalities and carries cultural connotations. Pious Christian nuns cover their hair. Muslim women wear headscarves to hide theirs from the eyes of all men but their husbands and immediate family. In India, hair is regarded as one of the most important aspects of feminine beauty. In some faiths, hair is cut during mourning. Several ancestral cultures still believe hair has magical powers; even in modern European countries some parents keep locks of their babies' hair.

Legends abound about hair: when Biblical hero Samson's long hair was cut, he lost his power; and, while blondes have more fun, redheads are believed to have a fiery temperament. Thankfully, many of these perceptions are not scientifically supported!

> *Assuming about 80 per cent of scalp hairs are in the active growth phase at any given time, a human produces about 9km (5.6 miles) of hair every year.*

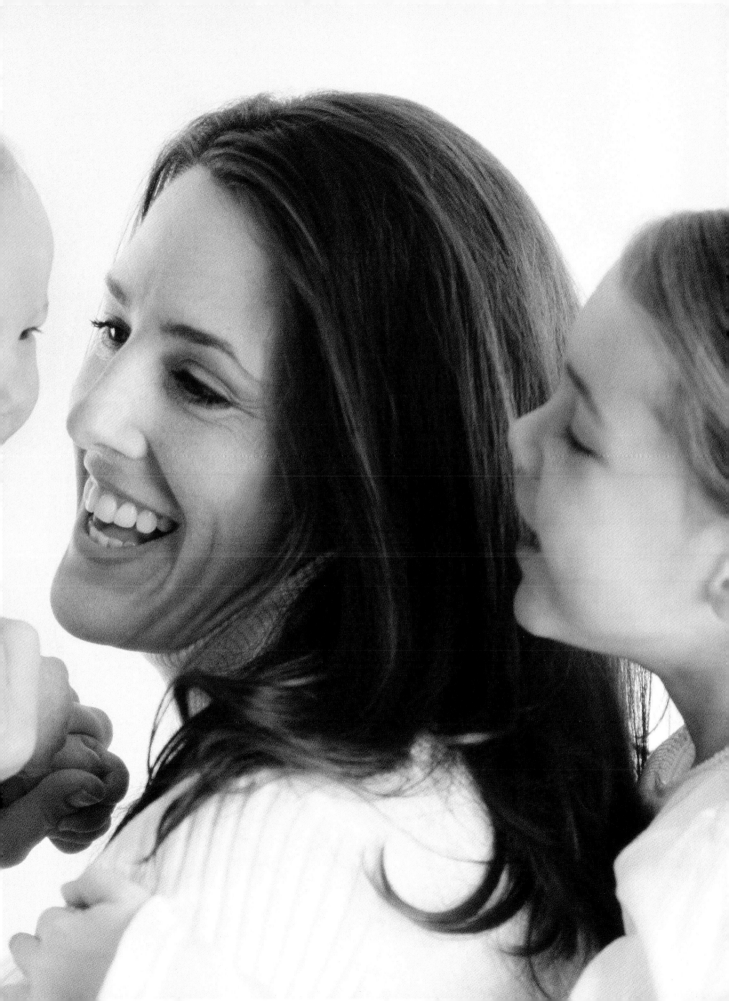

Your hair's structure

Given that healthy hair is a reflection of one's general health, it is ironic that the visible part of a hair – the hair shaft – is physiologically speaking, dead, with only the tiny part underneath the scalp (the root or dermal papilla) consisting of living hair-forming cells known as trichocytes and keratinocytes. The dermal papilla, nourished by a network of blood vessels and nerves, is nestled in a tubelike hair follicle and surrounded by what is known as the bulb. The bulb is embedded about 4mm (0.2in) in the subcutaneous fat of the scalp. The outer layers of the hair bulb are known as the outer and inner root sheaths. It is in the dermal papilla that most hair growth takes place. In order for hair to grow, cells have to reproduce. This takes place around the dermal papilla in what scientists call the zone of proliferation.

Each hair has a protective outer cuticle, made up of tiny overlapping scales, often compared to miniature roof tiles, and a thick cortex that lies under the cuticle and consists of the protein keratin. Keratin is also found in human skin and nails, as well as in the feathers, claws, hooves and wool of birds and animals.

Hair also contains the elements carbon, oxygen, nitrogen and sulphur and a tiny percentage of the trace elements zinc, iron, copper and iodine. Other components include fats, and water, which makes up about 12 per cent of a hair's weight.

Some types of hair – particularly thick, dark hair – also have a central medulla, which when inspected under an optical microscope, looks a little like a central canal. Some scientists believe it enhances the thermal-insulation properties of hair. Others speculate that the medulla carries nutrients to the cuticle and cortex, while yet another theory is that it contributes to the shine of hair.

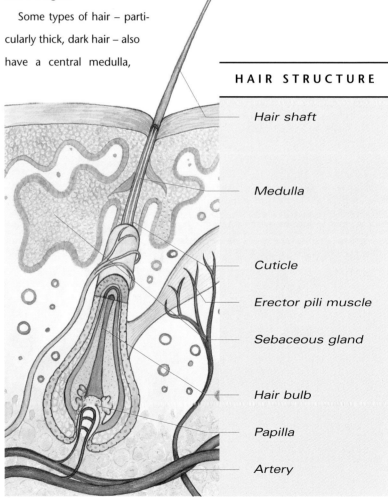

HAIR STRUCTURE

Hair shaft

Medulla

Cuticle

Erector pili muscle

Sebaceous gland

Hair bulb

Papilla

Artery

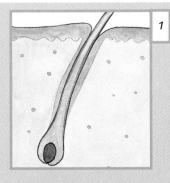

The anagen phase: Active growth takes place in the hair bulb. This phase can last for years, often between three and seven years.

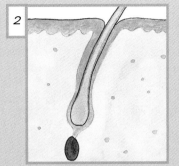

The catagen phase: This is a relatively short phase, during which the follicle stops producing hair and the hair bulb starts to break down.

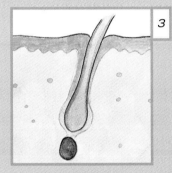

The telogen phase: A resting phase during which there is no growth and the hair is ready to be shed.

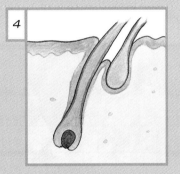

A new anagen phase: The old 'club hair' is ready to fall or be pushed out.

THE GROWTH CYCLE OF HAIR

Hair passes through a growth cycle broken up into three main phases: an active growth phase known as the anagen phase; a short, transitional catagen phase during which the hair stops growing and the hair bulb begins to break down (but there is still cellular activity in the papilla); and a resting telogen phase when no growth takes place and the hair is ready to be shed. The duration of the different phases varies from person to person, but the anagen phase can last anything from three to seven years, and in some cases even up to nine years. The catagen phase lasts roughly two to four weeks, while the telogen phase is estimated to last three to four months.

Function of the cortex and cuticle

The cortex cells give hair its strength and elasticity, while the cuticle reflects its condition.

If the protective scales of the cuticle are undamaged and lie flat, hair appears shiny and healthy, and is soft and manageable, but if they have been broken or damaged through straightening or colouring, hair looks dull and unhealthy. Environmental factors, including sunlight, air pollution and wind, can also damage the cuticle. The more damaged it is, the more tangled hair becomes and the more difficult it is to brush. Hair with smooth cuticle surfaces, on the other hand, reflects more light than hair with rough cuticle surfaces, which is why straight hair appears glossier than curly hair.

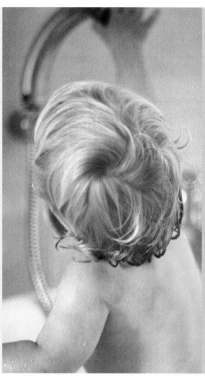

Different types of human hair

- **Lanugo hair** is the first hair to be produced by the hair follicles of a developing foetus. It normally covers the foetus until the seventh or eighth month of gestation, is fine and soft and contains no medulla and no pigment. After it has been shed, it is replaced by vellus hair and terminal hair.

- Newborn babies' bodies are covered with **vellus hair**, although they have terminal hair on their heads and eyebrows. The fine hair on parts of some adults' bodies is also vellus hair. These hairs are short, just a centimetre or two long, and they are soft, with no medulla. Occasionally, they contain pigment.

- **Terminal hair**, which grows on the head and also makes up beards, eyelashes and armpit hair, replaces vellus hair. These hairs are longer and coarser than vellus hair, often have a medulla and are usually pigmented.

A touch of colour

Melanin, found in the cortex, gives hair its colour. Pigment makes up only about one per cent of a hair, and although there is a wide range of human hair colours, they all derive from only two melanin pigments: eumelanin, a dark pigment predominating in black and brown hair, and phaeomelanin, a light pigment predominating in blonde and red hair. Many people's hair contains a mixture of the two pigments: the more eumelanin, the darker the hair.

Each hair has a tiny muscle – the erector pili – attached to it. This muscle contracts when it is cold, pulls the hair erect and causes goose flesh. Sebum, an oily substance secreted by the sebaceous glands in the skin, lubricates the hair, making it waterproof and shiny. As all teenagers discover sooner or later, an excess of sebum leads to greasy hair. Too little of it causes dry hair.

Thick or thin

We are all born with a set number of hair follicles and the thickness of our hair is determined by the size of these follicles: thick hair grows out of large follicles, while fine hair grows out of small follicles. So, unfortunately, there is no product on earth that can make your hair thicker or increase the number of hair follicles on your head! A single hair might appear thin and fragile, but according to international cosmetics giant L'Oréal, tests have shown that a healthy hair can carry a weight of about 100g (0.2 lb). If you multiply this by 120 000 – the average number of hairs on the human head – you can deduce that a head of hair could, theoretically, support 12 tonnes (in reality, of course, the scalp is not strong enough to make this possible).

The growth factor

Just like there are changes to the body and skin, your hair's structure and its appearance also change as you grow older.

■ Babies are born with a specific, genetically determined number of hair follicles. Yet some babies have hardly any hair at birth, while others have quite a bit. This is no indication of what the state of their hair will be later in life!

■ Small children's hair often has characteristics that are lost later in life. For example, blonde hair may darken as they grow older and curls may disappear. The thickness of children's hair increases fast until the age of three or four. The diameter continues to increase more slowly until the age of 10 or 11, when the hair should be at its thickest.

■ In puberty, the body undergoes a number of metabolic changes. These also affect the hair. The sebaceous glands are stimulated, often secreting an excess of oil and resulting in oily hair. Dandruff can also appear at this stage, the result of oil secretion and hormonal changes.

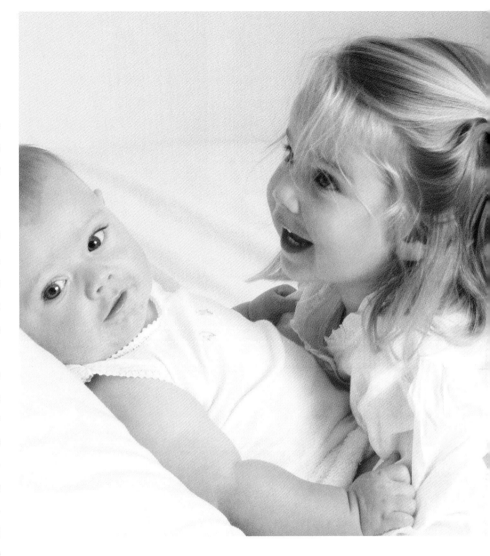

▲
This baby's sparse hair is no indication of what her hair might look like in future, and her sister may still find her blonde hair darkening.

■ Around the age of 25, the diameter of hair starts to decrease. In the next 15 years the hair-growth cycle changes, with fewer hairs in the anagen phase and more in the resting phase. Hair growth thus slows down.

■ The age at which grey hairs start appearing is genetically determined. Hair turns white when melanin is no longer produced. Individual hairs become thinner. Many men start losing their hair, and a percentage of women experiences some thinning.

Defining your ethnic hair type

Human hair – which grows everywhere on the body except the palms of the hands, soles of the feet, eyelids and lips – can differ markedly in texture and colour. Yet all human hair has similar functions. Scalp and body hair is believed to keep us warm by preserving heat. It cushions our heads, giving some protection against injury. The hair inside our nose and ears and around our eyes protects against dust and germs, while eyebrows and eyelashes protect our eyes against sweat, harsh light and tiny particles. Armpit hair helps to reduce friction.

Unlike other mammals, humans do not moult, because our hair follicles are all at different stages of the growth cycle at any given time. (If they had all been synchronized, everybody would have gone bald from time to time.) Nevertheless, we do shed our hair at a rate of 50 to 80 scalp hairs a day (the figure of 100 hairs a day, often quoted as the average daily hair loss, is now believed to be exaggerated). As we'll see later, factors like changing hormone levels, diet and medication can influence the hair-loss rate quite drastically.

Your hair type is determined by your genetic make-up; you can change your look, but not your hair's inherent characteristics.

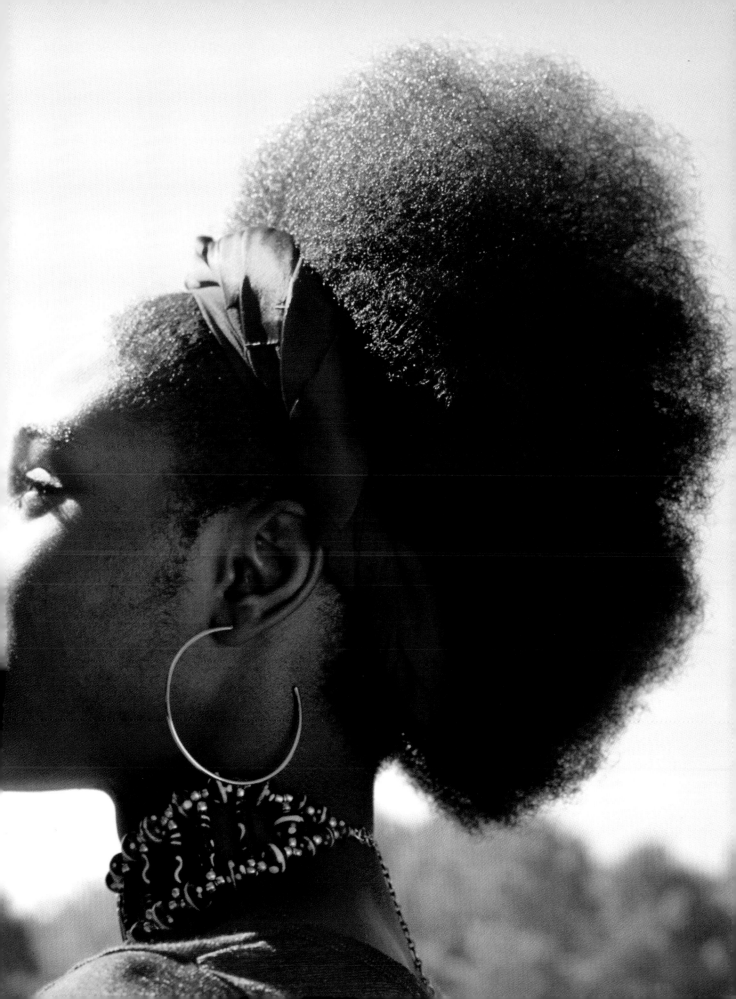

In a class of its own

Human hair can be coarse and black, fair and fine, straight and thick, wavy or kinky, but despite the different variations in colour and texture, it is generally classified into three ethnic types: Caucasian, Asian and African.

Although the hair of most Scandinavians differs markedly from that of a South American or Spaniard, they all have hair that can be classified as Caucasian. The same goes for Indonesian and Japanese hair – both are Asian hair types. Typical Caribbean hair is classified as African hair. Even though there are variations within hair types, the three main ethnic classifications have very distinctive characteristics.

Your hair type is determined by your genetic make-up and although there are ways to temporarily change its look, you can never change its inherent characteristics.

CHANGING YOUR LOOK

Unlike facial features or body shape, hair is relatively easy to change, and the hair products industry is booming, with industry players spending millions on research each year. A crucial element to offering consumers what they want and need is a thorough understanding of hair types.

The chemical compositions of the three ethnic hair types, and the molecular structure of the keratin therein, are all similar, but the hair shafts differ. While there is some understanding of the reasons for this, research into the differences continues.

African hair is dark and tightly curled; Asian hair tends to be straight, coarse, dark and thick, while Caucasian hair ranges from fine and straight to relatively thick and wavy, and has the greatest variation in colour. The differences between the hair types, according to international hair products company Wella, centre on its longitudinal and cross-sectional shape, thickness, ellipticity (whether the hair is 'round' or 'flat') and colour.

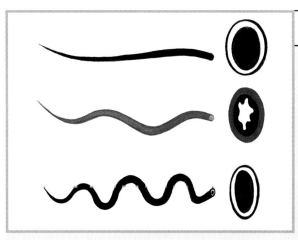

Axial shapes   Ellipticity

HOW HAIR TYPES DIFFER IN SHAPE

◀ *Asian hair: This hair type has an approximately round shape.*

◀ *Caucasian: This hair type has an oval shape.*

◀ *African: This hair type is extremely oval, almost flat.*

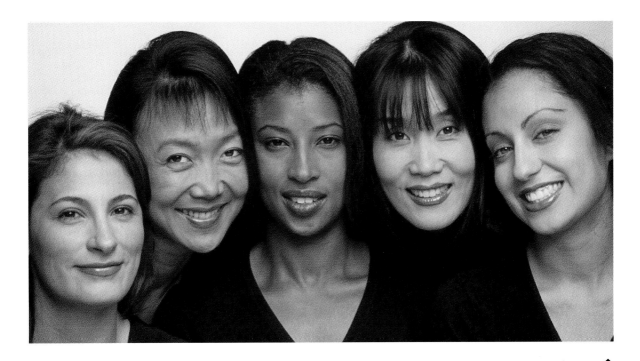

Texture

A strand of Caucasian hair has an average thickness of 0.07mm (3in) and, seen in cross section, has an oval shape. Coarser Asian hair, about 0.09mm (3.5in) thick, has an approximately round shape, while African hair, ranging between 0.04 (1.6in) and 0.12mm (5in) in thickness, is extremely oval (nearly 'flat').

It is generally no longer believed that the shape of a curly hair is caused by a curved hair follicle. The follicles of curly hair are, in fact, straight. Further evidence that follicle shape has nothing to do with the curliness or straightness of hair is that some types of medication may cause curly hair to suddenly go straight, without any change to the follicle. All hair – even straight Asian hair – twists as it grows, but the more it twists, the curlier it is. African hair is the most fragile of the three hair types.

Hair product company L'Oréal's institute for ethnic hair and skin research considers the particular structure of African hair to be the reason for this. As mentioned, each African hair shaft has a distinct oval – almost flat – shape. The outer cuticle scales protecting each hair are thinner in the areas where the oval-shaped hair shaft is thinnest. As a result, these thin parts of the cuticle

An example of typical Caucasian, African and Asian hair types. Caucasian hair has the greatest variation in texture and colour.

break easily, exposing the inner cortex of the hair. Once the more vulnerable cortex is no longer protected it then also breaks easily. In addition, the chemical composition of a part of the cuticle, prone to microscopic cracks, causes African hair to have weak mechanical resistance, according to L'Oréal scientists.

The weak points along the hair shaft and the spiral twists make African hair quite difficult to groom, and certainly more difficult to comb than straight Caucasian hair. It is also more brittle, splits more easily and has a lower moisture content. To straighten such hair, heavy-duty chemicals are needed, and damage is bound to occur to the hair structure.

Asian hair is thicker than Caucasian hair and has about 10 layers of cuticle cells, making it stronger and stiffer with more body. Asian hair contains a medulla filled with plenty of dark pigment, thought to contribute to their shine and high moisture content. Asian hair also tends to grow longer than African and Caucasian hair as it has the longest growth cycle of the three hair types: up to nine years. In addition it grows faster than African and Caucasian hair – about 1.3cm (0.5in) per month, compared to the

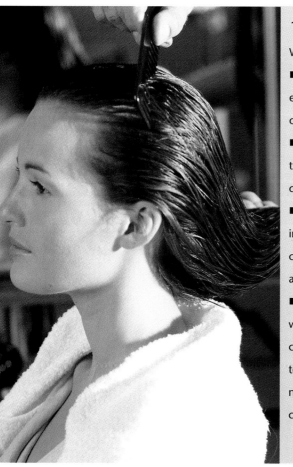

The characteristics of hair

Whatever your hair type, all hair shares certain properties:

■ It is elastic because of the coiled structure of the keratin, and this elasticity increases when hair is wet. Because of its elasticity, a healthy hair can stretch up to 20 or 30 per cent of its length before it breaks.

■ Hair swells (gets thicker) if it is soaked in water, as the water enters the air spaces between the fibres of the cortex. A hair in good condition can, in fact, absorb about 30 per cent of its own weight in water.

■ Hair is porous, and liquids can pass between the outer cuticle scales into the cortex. Porosity increases if the cuticle is damaged or if the cuticle scales are lifted through heat, steam or chemical treatments. Sebum and certain conditioning creams or lacquers can decrease the porosity.

■ Hair is hygroscopic and absorbs moisture from the air. This explains why the same head of hair can behave very differently in dry and humid conditions. When it is humid, hair absorbs a lot more moisture and tends to become frizzy, whereas it tends to be straight in a dry climate. The normal moisture content of hair is about 10 per cent of its weight, but this can increase to 30 per cent.

1.2cm (0.4in) and 0.9cm (3.5in) of the two other hair types respectively. On average, Asians also shed fewer hairs a day than Africans or Caucasians, and Asian men tend to experience less balding (Caucasians have the highest incidence of male-pattern baldness).

Greying also starts later. However, there is evidence that Asian women over 45 tend to experience more overall thinning of hair than their Caucasian and African counterparts, and because Asian hair is thicker and often longer than other hair types it tends to lose more moisture, which leads to dryness and split ends.

About 70 per cent of Caucasians have finely textured hair, and 30 per cent have medium-textured or coarse hair. Colour and texture appear to be linked: blondes tend to have the finest hair, while redheads tend to have the coarsest. Although Asian hair is thicker, Caucasian hair has the highest density of the three hair types.

Hair can be fine, medium-textured or coarse. Fine hair always tends to lack volume, while medium hair is often quite easy to handle, strong and elastic. Coarse hair brings its own problems: it is abundant, but can be heavy, frizzy and difficult to control. You may find that you have fine hair in your hairline and on your temples, while the rest of your hair is medium or coarse.

A QUESTION OF OIL AND MOISTURE

Whether you have dry, oily, normal or combination hair depends on how much oil your sebaceous glands produce, and how you treat your hair. It is impossible to stop your sebaceous glands producing grease, and it is also an old wives' tale that oil production is very much affected by your diet. Eating too many chocolates or greasy food may well lead to weight gain, but it will not make your hair oilier! While you cannot change your genetics, understanding your hair type and treating it accordingly can help you have a healthy, good-looking head of hair.

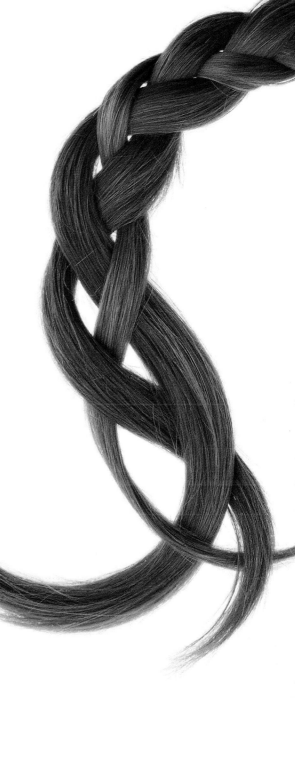

Oily hair

If your sebaceous glands produce too much sebum, your scalp and hair tend to be oily and your hair may even become lank and greasy only a few hours after you have washed it. You will therefore need to wash it more often than someone with normal hair. Contrary to popular belief, frequent washing does not exacerbate the oil problem. If you tend to have greasy hair, do not touch it often or run your fingers through it constantly, as this can make hair appear greasy quicker. Too much brushing also helps to distribute oil. While some experts advise using a shampoo formulated for oily hair, others believe that it's better to wash your hair often with a mild shampoo. Apply conditioner only to the ends. A good tip is to use hairspray after you have styled your hair. This keeps it out of your face and stops you from touching it frequently.

Dry hair

Dry hair – which literally contains too little moisture – can be caused by a variety of factors: naturally it is the result of sebaceous glands producing too little sebum, but chemical treatments, frequent washing, harsh sunlight, wind, overuse of hair-dryers and hair age (hair that has not been cut for a long time) can also cause dry, brittle hair. This hair type can lack shine, feel rough and break, and

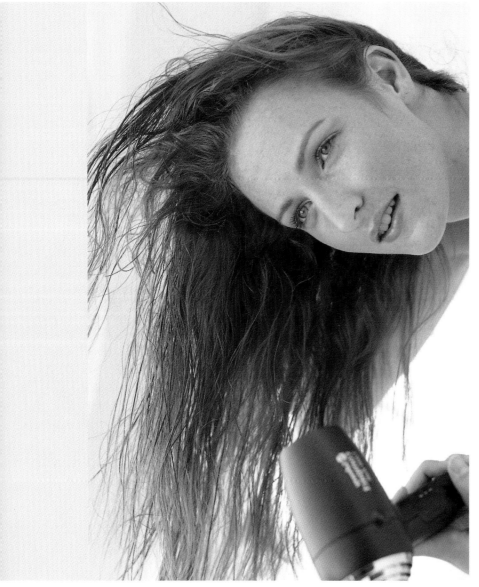

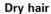 *Heat from a hair-dryer can be damaging to hair. Try to cut down on blow-drying, particularly if your hair tends to be dry and brittle.*

tangle easily. Use a shampoo for dry hair and always follow a wash with conditioner. Try to cut down on blow-drying and avoid chemical treatments such as bleaching, straightening and perming. A regular hot-oil treatment may help, but the better solution for dry and split ends is to cut them off.

Normal hair

Normal hair is neither too dry nor too oily, feels soft and healthy and does not tangle easily. This type of hair is easy to manage and style, and usually has not been coloured, straightened or permed. The sebaceous glands tend to produce just the right amount of oil, but a healthy lifestyle, qood qroominq habits and sensible treatment of your hair also help. Wash your hair regularly, but not every day, and use a light conditioner.

Combination hair

If your roots and scalp are oily, but your hair ends are dry, you have combination hair. This can be the result of treatments which strip the hair of moisture. Harsh sunlight and long hair that has not been cut for some time can also lead to combination hair. When washing your hair, concentrate on the scalp area and always use moisturizing conditioner on the ends. Bear in mind the guidelines for both oily and dry hair if you have combination hair: do not touch your hair too much, and go easy on the hair-dryer and styling tools.

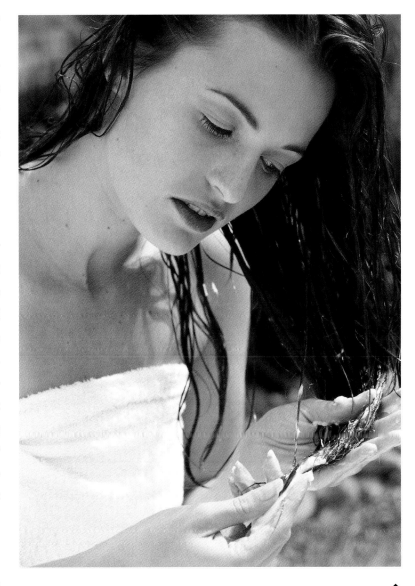

▲

The only cure for split ends is to cut them off, but conditioner can help to prevent further damage and improve the feel of your hair.

Hair and scalp problems

Although the visible part of each hair on your body is, technically speaking, dead your hair is still one of the best barometers of your general health and one of the quickest indicators that something is wrong. This is because hair-forming cells in the dermal papilla are some of the fastest dividing cells in the human body. Baldness and thinning hair affect millions of people and can be hereditary, or caused by a variety of factors.

A loss in the condition of your hair can be an early warning sign of an underlying problem. See a doctor if you notice flaking, itching or crusting of the scalp, a sudden increased hair loss – particularly if accompanied by other symptoms – and irritated skin patches on the scalp. Unfortunately, not all remedies on the market are based on scientific principles, so make sure you get an authoritative medical view before trying a new treatment. Also, not all hair problems make sense – sometimes even the most experienced specialist will not be able to pinpoint the reason for hair loss, for example.

Be aware that a loss in the condition of your hair can be an early warning sign of an underlying problem.

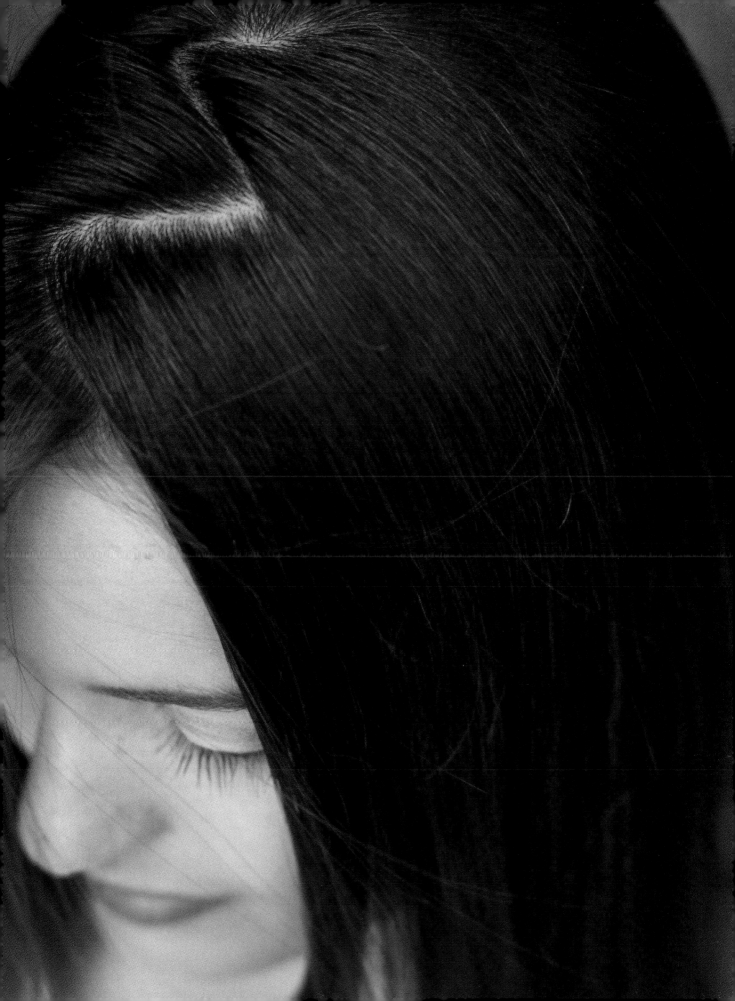

Hair loss

Hair loss (alopecia) can affect anyone – man, woman or child – at any time, but male-pattern hair loss or male androgenetic alopecia is the most common form.

It is normal to lose between 50 and 80 hairs daily but when the hairs you are losing start to outnumber the new hairs appearing, your hair will start thinning; if this continues, you will start balding. There are a number of treatments available, but their efficacy depends on the type of hair loss you are experiencing.

MALE- AND FEMALE- PATTERN HAIR LOSS

Male-pattern hair loss is the most common type of hair loss in men and is usually hereditary – a history of androgenetic alopecia on either side of the family increases a man's risk of balding. Heredity also affects the age at which men begin to lose hair, as well as the speed and extent of the loss.

Male-pattern baldness usually starts with a receding hairline, leading to baldness on the top of the head, which then spreads. Hair loss can start any time after puberty. Caucasian men are more likely to lose hair than African or Asian men – it is estimated that 96 per cent of mature Caucasian men experience some recession in their hairline, even if they are not destined to lose all their hair. Male-pattern hair loss is discussed in more detail in Chapter 8.

Although androgenetic alopecia mostly affects men, some women also get it. It is then called female-pattern hair loss, or female-pattern androgenetic alopecia. The pattern differs from the male hair-loss pattern in that the woman's hairline does not recede, rather the hair

Stress and hair loss

It is believed that there is a link between stress and depression, and hair loss. There are documented cases of people starting to lose hair, anything from a few weeks to a few months after a stressful episode in their lives. Of course, hair loss itself is stressful, so it is not always clear which came first, hair loss or stress.

According to the American Academy of Dermatology, men and women with androgenetic alopecia have a higher incidence of personality disorders. According to the academy, women with hair loss experience a lack of self-esteem, are introverted, feel less attractive, and are tense in public places.

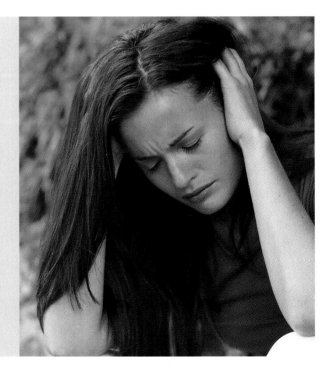

becomes thin over the entire scalp. Women suffering from female-pattern hair loss are likely to first notice it somewhere between their late 20s and early 40s. They are particularly prone to some hair loss at times of hormonal change, for example when they start or stop taking the contraceptive pill, after having a baby and during early menopause.

Handle thinning hair gently: avoid overbrushing and steer clear of appliances or hair tools that pull the hair. Granny's advice was well meant, but 100 strokes a day will do more bad than good.

Alopecia areata

Alopecia areata – which can cause all, or much, of the hair on the head or body to fall out – is thought to affect about two per cent of the population in some form, at some point in their lives. Some people only experience one small patch of hair loss, while others may have many large patches.

Alopecia areata is classified as an autoimmune disease – the result of the immune system's white blood cells attacking the fast-growing hair cells in the follicles. No-one knows what causes the white blood cells to do this. As a result, the follicles

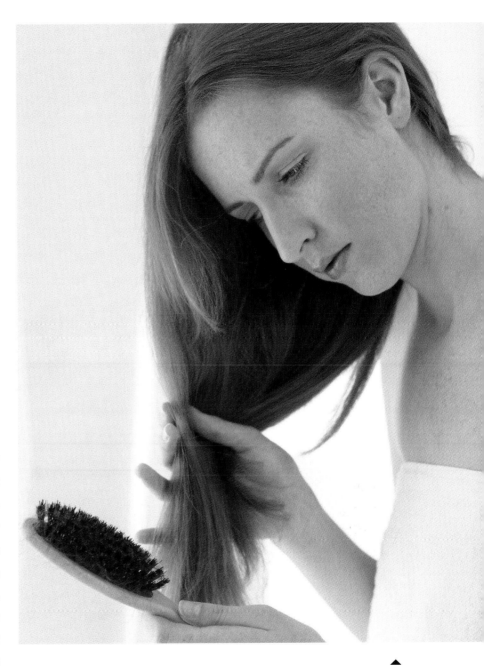

▲

Always handle your hair gently. Use a quality hairbrush and do not over-brush or pull on your tresses.

become smaller and hair production slows down. The hairs that are produced are fragile and break off even before they reach the skin's surface. Alopecia areata is a very distressing condition, but fortunately often disappears as suddenly as it appears. Alopecia areata does not cause follicles to lose the potential to form new hair, but hair may take years to grow back. Some scientists believe certain people may be genetically predisposed to it.

There are different types of alopecia areata: if all your scalp hair, as well as your eyebrows and eyelashes fall out, this condition is known as alopecia areata totalis. When all the hair on your head, face, and body is lost, the condition is known as alopecia areata universalis.

There is no cure for alopecia areata, but certain treatments – including cortisone injections or pills – may alleviate the condition. Tarlike ointments, commonly used to treat the skin disease psoriasis, may stimulate new hair growth.

Disease

If your thyroid gland is overactive or underactive, your hair may fall out. When the thyroid disease is treated, the hair-loss problem is usually solved. An overactive thyroid (hyperthyroidism) may lead to scalp hair becoming fine and soft with some hair loss, while an underactive thyroid (hypothyroidism) can lead to dry, coarse head and body hair, and partial hair loss.

Many chronic illnesses, including bowel disorders involving malabsorption, endocrine abnormalities, renal and hepatic disease and cancer (even without chemotherapy) are also associated with hair loss. Conditions like diabetes and the autoimmune disease lupus may also cause hair loss.

Hormone imbalance and childbirth

If male hormones (androgens) or female hormones (oestrogens) are out of balance, it can lead to hair loss. Correcting the imbalance may stop your hair loss. Some types of birth-control pills – particularly the older types – may also lead to hair loss for some women.

Many women shed quite a lot of hair for several months after having a baby. This commonly starts about three months after the birth and is nothing to worry about. It is also related to hormonal changes in

It is a myth that...

■   shampoos and conditioners can cause abnormal hair loss. This is rarely, if ever, the case.

■   hair can turn white overnight. In fact, the greying process is gradual. (Sufferers of alopecia areata, however, may find that their regrowing hairs are white, which may have led to this myth.)

■   dandruff is infectious, or the result of bad hygiene or stress. Not true.

■   baldness is inherited from the mother's family. It can be inherited from your mother or father's side of the family, but sometimes there is no history of baldness on either side of the family, and you are simply unlucky!

■   vitamins and proteins can be absorbed into hair. This is impossible; the only way they can benefit your hair is through a healthy diet.

the body. During pregnancy, the hair-growth cycle changes and far fewer hairs are shed than normally, the result of high oestrogen levels that keep hairs in the active growing phase. Following the baby's birth, oestrogen levels return to pre-pregnancy levels, more hairs go into the resting telogen phase and are shed as the growth cycle returns to normal.

Medication and medical treatment

Certain drugs may cause hair loss. These include particular medications for gout, arthritis, depression, heart problems and high blood pressure. If you stop the medication, your hair should grow back, or the doctor may be able to prescribe an alternative that does not have this side effect.

Chemotherapy often causes hair loss, because it targets fast-growing cancer cells and, as a consequence, also affects fast-growing hair cells. Hair loss – which does not always start immediately – can occur on all parts of the body. The hair usually grows back after the treatments are over. Sometimes, hair may grow back a different colour or texture. Special ice caps, to be worn during chemotherapy sessions, may improve your chances of keeping your hair.

Fever or surgery

You may find yourself losing more hair than normal two to five months after an illness accompanied by a prolonged fever. Scientists believe the cause is hair entering its telogen phase early. The situation normally rectifies itself. You may also lose some hair after an operation, although the reason for this has not been established.

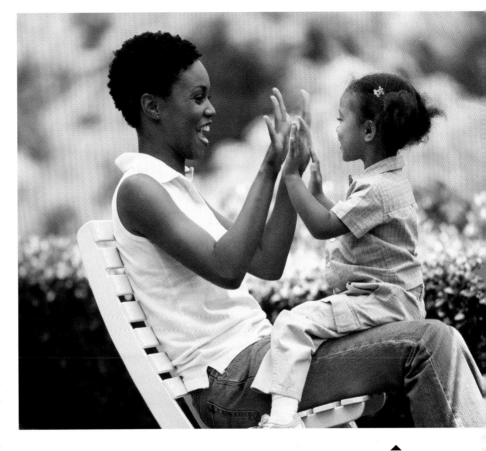

▲

Many women lose quite a lot of hair in the months following the birth of a baby, but the situation normally rectifies itself without medical intervention.

Scalp disorders

The scalp differs from the skin on your body in that it has an abundant supply of oil from the sebaceous glands and has hair follicles that produce long terminal hair. Most scalp problems are easy to solve, others are chronic and more problematic.

DANDRUFF

Dandruff (*pityriasis simplex* or *furfuracea*) is more of an aesthetic concern than a medical problem. It has been associated with a tiny yeast cell (*Pityrosporum ovale*) found on all scalps, but which seems to grow more rapidly on the heads of dandruff sufferers. Dandruff has a social stigma, and sufferers dread the sight of the characteristic small white scales – tiny pieces of skin shed from the scalp. Dandruff is more common in men than women, suggesting there is some link with male androgens.

By the age of 20, about half of all Caucasians are affected by dandruff to some degree, and the condition often clears spontaneously by 50 or 60 years of age. There are many effective antidandruff shampoos on the market, but the scales normally

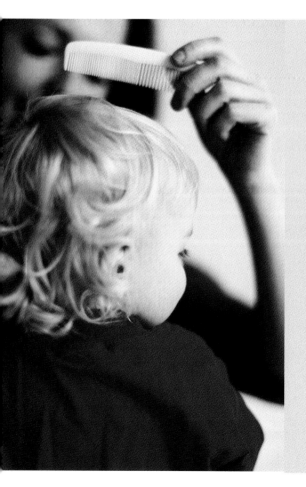

Common scalp infections

Even in First World countries, infections by fungi, bacteria and lice – collectively known as dermatophytes – are fairly common. These organisms are transferred quite easily through personal contact and shared towels, bedding and clothing.

One of the most common scalp infections is scalp ringworm, or *tinea capitis*. This fungal infection causes itchy, circular patches on the skin and can lead to some hair loss. It is easily spread – not only on combs or brushes but even on furniture. Ringworm, which mostly affects children, can be treated with antifungals and lost hair generally grows back once the infection is under control.

Head lice (*pediculosis capitis* or *pediculosis*) – identified by an itchy scalp and eggs attached to hair roots – are transmitted through contact with clothes and grooming tools. Infection has nothing to do with hygiene, dirty hair or personal grooming habits. In fact, lice love long, clean hair! Although treatments are available, studies suggest lice are becoming resistant to the products. Experts believe that removal using a nit comb is still the most effective.

form again within four to seven days. It's a good idea to alternate a dandruff shampoo with a regular shampoo (although antidandruff shampoos are generally not harsher on hair than other shampoos). Effective antidandruff ingredients include zinc pyrithione, salicylic acid compounds, selenium sulfide or coal tar (in small concentrations).

SEBORRHOEA

Seborrhoea is characterized by a very greasy scalp and greasy hair. It has also been linked with hirsutism (excessive facial and body hair). The condition can quite effectively be controlled with specially formulated shampoos.

Seborrhoeic dermatitis is more serious. It is a form of chronic eczema resembling psoriasis and is characterized by large, greasy yellow scales. It is not known what causes it. Seborrhoeic dermatitis can be treated with corticosteroid lotions and antifungal shampoos.

PSORIASIS

This disorder is often not confined to the scalp, but its effects on the scalp include silvery scales and tender, sometimes itchy, skin. Treatments include tar-based shampoos, salicylic acid, cortisone and ultraviolet light.

ECZEMA

Eczema affects different parts of the body, including sometimes the scalp, and causes itching and soreness. There is no cure for it, although some treatments alleviate the symptoms.

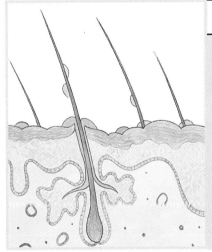

CONTACT DERMATITIS

As the name suggests, this condition flares up on contact with a product – such as a hair colourant or straightening solution – that the scalp is sensitive or allergic to. If your skin flares up after using a certain product, switch to another, preferably with less colouring or perfume.

SEBORRHOEA

Seborrhoea, characterized by abnormal secretions of the sebaceous glands, can be controlled with medicated shampoo.

DANDRUFF

Dandruff is a common condition leading to small white scales (tiny pieces of skin) being shed from the scalp.

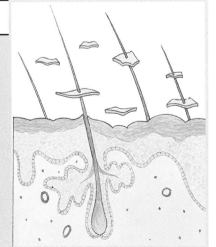

Treatment for hair loss

Treatment depends on the cause and extent of your hair loss, and contrary to claims by many marketers keen to exploit those desperate to reverse their natural hair loss, there simply is no magic cure.

One of the most well-known treatments for hair loss, approved by the United States Food and Drug Administration and other regulatory bodies, is the drug **minoxidil** (available over the counter as Rogaine™ or Regaine™).

A side effect of minoxidil, which was originally used to treat hypertension, is increased hair growth. It is available in two and five per cent solutions and is rubbed topically on to the scalp. Some users do seem to experience some regrowth, but the new hair is often thinner and lighter and dryness or irritation of the scalp may be experienced. Unfortunately, minoxidil does not work for everybody and commonly appears only to slow down the rate of hair loss.

Another drawback is that new growth ceases as soon as users stop taking the drug – and its prolonged use could get very expensive.

Another drug that has been shown to slow hair loss and bring about some new hair growth is **finasteride**, marketed as Propecia™.

Modern hair-implant methods – ▶
using mini and micro grafts – yield
better results than older methods
and also give a more natural
regrowth pattern.

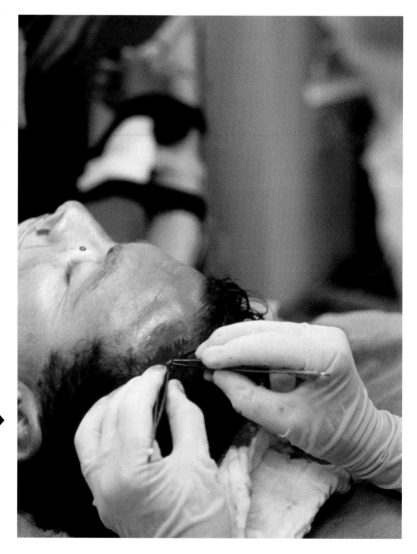

This medication, taken in tablet form, is only used for male-pattern baldness and is not approved for use by women as its suitability during pregnancy has not been established.

The drug works in men by inhibiting the conversion of testosterone into dihydrotestosterone, a hormone significant in male hair loss, as it shrinks hair follicles. Side effects are rare, but research suggests it can temporarily affect sexual function or libido in about two per cent of users. Again, benefits cease once the drug is stopped.

Neither minoxidil nor finasteride should be used for hair loss due to illness.

Hair-implantation methods have improved in recent years, with mini and micro hair grafts yielding better results than the older punch-biopsy methods that often failed. Modern hair grafts also give a more natural regrowth pattern. (*See* Chapter 8 for more about surgical solutions to hair loss.)

Hair-loss fact file

- By the age of 50, half of all men will have some obvious hair loss.
- Hair loss starts an average of 10 years later in women than in men.
- Humans are not the only mammals to suffer from baldness. Chimpanzees and orang-utans often also show signs of baldness when they reach sexual maturity.
- Women's hairlines tend to remain unchanged throughout life even though they may experience general thinning, but about half of all men can expect their hairline to recede to some extent as they get older.
- Many alcoholics experience poor hair growth, or even hair loss, as their illness can lead to malnutrition.
- Trichotillomania is a compulsive desire to pull out one's own hair. This habit can lead to damage of the hair root (if the hairs are pulled out during the active anagen growth phase). Trichotillomania seems to be more common in women than in men, and children can also suffer from it.

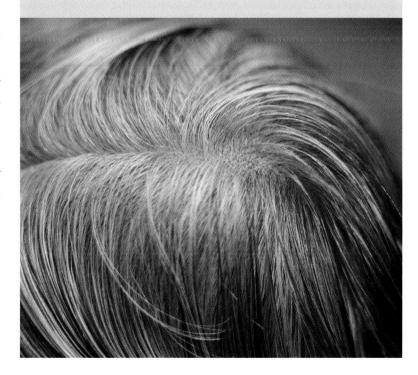

The impact of diet

Growing hair receives nourishment by means of the bloodstream and, contrary to claims by some manufacturers, products applied to the hair externally cannot nourish it, although they may improve the hair's condition.

A healthy diet is therefore important for hair health.

Protein is vital for building hair but increasing the amount of protein in the diet does not necessarily increase hair growth. Malnutrition, or a serious lack of protein in your diet, can lead to hair loss. The condition known as Protein Energy Malnutrition not only leads to hair loss but also causes dry, brittle hair.

According to the American Academy of Dermatology, calorie and/or protein malnutrition forces the body to save protein by shifting growing hairs into the resting phase. This causes shedding of the hair spread out over the entire scalp. This type of hair loss, known as telogen effluvium, is slow and often not noticeable until nearly half the hair is lost. Body hair, on the other hand, may increase at the same time. By returning to a balanced diet, the hair loss can be reversed.

While it is well known that one of the noticeable manifestations of the eating disorder anorexia nervosa is hair loss, dieters often do not realize that

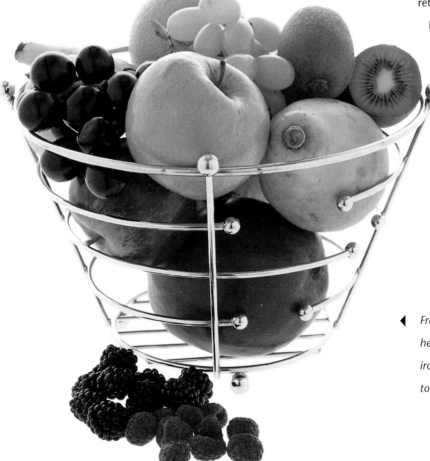

◀ *Fresh fruit contains Vitamin C, which helps with the absorption of iron (and iron deficiency and anaemia can lead to hair loss).*

Hair analysis - a far-fetched fad?

Hair analysis involves the testing of hair strands to confirm the presence or absence of specific substances. Practitioners promoting hair analysis claim that the levels of minerals in the hair correlate with the levels in the body, and that by testing hair they can check for deficiencies (or abnormally high quantities) of minerals in the body. Many then offer supplements to address these deficiencies.

Scientists tend to be sceptical about these claims, however, and many believe them to be unreliable. Scientific studies have concluded that analysis is not particularly useful for assessing levels of minerals such as sodium, magnesium, phosphorus, potassium, calcium, iron and iodine in the body. Researchers have also pointed out that dyes, chemical treatments, age, season and hair length, may affect the results. It is, therefore, unlikely that nutritional therapy based on hair analysis is of any benefit, and it is more than likely a waste of your money. What's more, instances have been recorded where different laboratories came to different conclusions after testing identical hair samples!

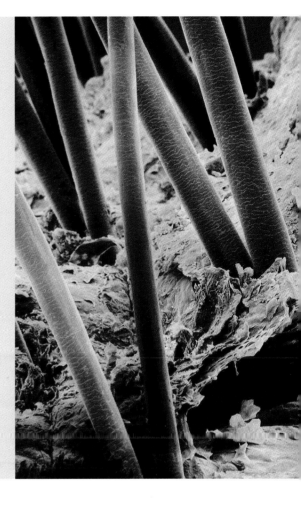

they do not have to be noticeably underweight, or suffer from an eating disorder to start losing hair. In fact, dieticians have noticed that a loss of a mere five kilograms (11 lb) can lead to some hair loss, particularly if you cut down drastically on protein and/or fats.

As a diet high in fat poses health risks, try to choose mainly low-fat proteins such as fish, chicken, lean red meat, eggs, milk and pulses. Make sure you eat enough food containing vitamins and minerals. It is important to eat enough sources of Vitamin C (available from fresh fruit and vegetables) and Vitamin B (found in oily fish, peas, eggs, milk and wholegrain cereals) on a daily basis. The Vitamin B complex, and particularly biotin, is important to keep hair follicles in good health. It appears that a lack of biotin (found in nuts and eggs) may lead to a reduction in activity in hair follicles. Vitamin B1 is also believed to be important for healthy hair. (Even so, there is no proof that taking Vitamin-B supplements actually prevents hair loss.)

Although Vitamin C cannot be directly linked to healthy hair, it does help with absorption of iron (iron deficiency and anaemia can lead to

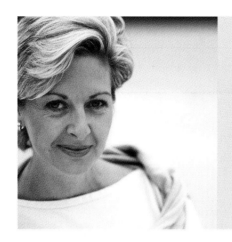

A grey matter

Greying is not a medical problem, but a natural process. Cells in the dermal papilla manufacture hair pigment (melanin). As you grow older these cells make less pigment. The result is grey hair that still contains some pigment and, ultimately, white hair that has none at all. The age at which you start greying and the rate at which grey hairs appear depend on genetic factors.

hair loss). Telogen effluvium which results from an iron deficiency is relatively common in young women who menstruate. Doctors do not always pick this up, since they may test for aneamia and the result may come back negative. Make sure that your iron stores, in particular, are checked if you suspect that your levels are low. Also ensure that your diet contains enough iron-rich foods, including green leafy vegetables, eggs, dates, raisins and liver (but avoid liver if you are pregnant, as it contains very high concentrations of Vitamin A, which can harm the developing foetus).

In large doses, Vitamin A causes hair loss, and some drugs that contain

Save your hair

Do an Internet search, or visit health shops and pharmacies, and you will find many products claiming to combat hair loss. In truth, very few of these can promote hair growth or stop hair loss.

In 1980, an advisory panel to the US Food and Drug Administration studied a number of substances that are used in hair-growth products. They found them to be ineffective and proposed that they be removed from the market.

The substances included jojoba oil, lanolin and wheat-germ oil, which are often said to combat alopecia. Others on the list were amino acids, amino-benzoic acid, ascorbic acid, benzoic acid, B vitamins, hormones, sulphanilamide and tetracaine hydrochloride, as well as urea.

Scalp massage, changes in diet (unless you had an eating disorder or were seriously malnourished), electrical stimulation and Chinese herbal extracts are not effective tools to treat androgenetic alopecia either. Similarly, vasodilators – products that you rub into the scalp, supposedly to increase and stimulate blood supply and hair growth – are also a waste of money.

Vitamin A derivatives are also associated with this problem. Such drugs inhibit cell division and slow down keratinization, thereby slowing down activity in the hair follicles.

Hereditary or acquired zinc deficiency is also known to lead to hair loss, so make sure you have enough zinc in your diet (found in shellfish, red meat and pumpkin seeds). Zinc can improve thyroid function (and an underactive thyroid, as mentioned, may lead to thinning hair).

Supplements that can improve the condition of your hair in the long term include those containing essential fatty acids such as flaxseed and evening primrose oil. Essential fatty acids are also found in oily fish and nuts.

It makes sense that a well-balanced diet, which is good for your body, is also good for your hair. Drink at least eight glasses of water a day. Finally, since your hair follicles need a good supply of oxygen and nutrients from the blood, it cannot hurt to boost your circulation with exercise! However, it has to be stressed that boosting your circulation alone will unfortunately not lead to your hair growing faster or thicker.

Plenty of water and exercise is good for your general health and thus for your hair.

▼

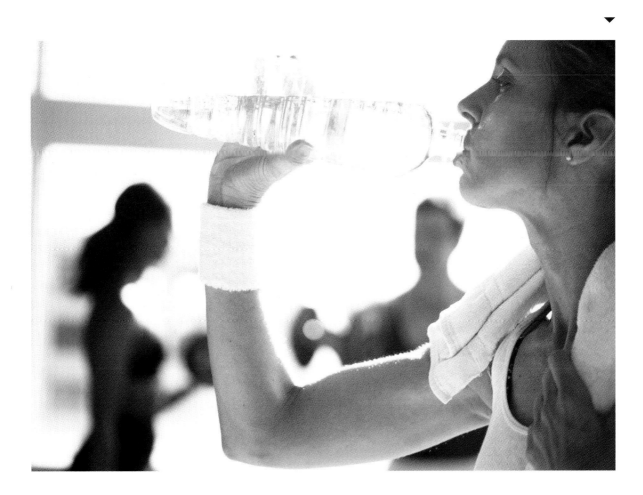

Treatments, tools & tackle

A bottle of shampoo might be the most basic hair grooming product in any bathroom today, but this has not always been the case: in the 17th and 18th centuries, most people did not wash their hair more than once or twice a year. Marie Antoinette, the self-indulgent last queen of France, and her peers are said to have used perfumes, potpourri and perfumed candles in a desperate attempt to disguise the resultant odours. To compound the problem, high-society ladies wore such elaborate hairstyles that many would spend nights sleeping sitting up rather than risk ruining their crowning glories. Elaborate hair constructions built over wire cages were decorated not only with feathers and jewels, but even fruit, vegetables and animal menageries, attracting rats and other vermin.

You should wash your hair as often as needed. Washing it daily will not trigger your sebaceous glands to produce more oil.

Fortunately we no longer need smelling salts to cope with our lack of sensible hair hygiene. The menageries are out of fashion, but our hairstyle choices still say a lot about who we are, and the myriad treatments and products on the market bear testimony to this.

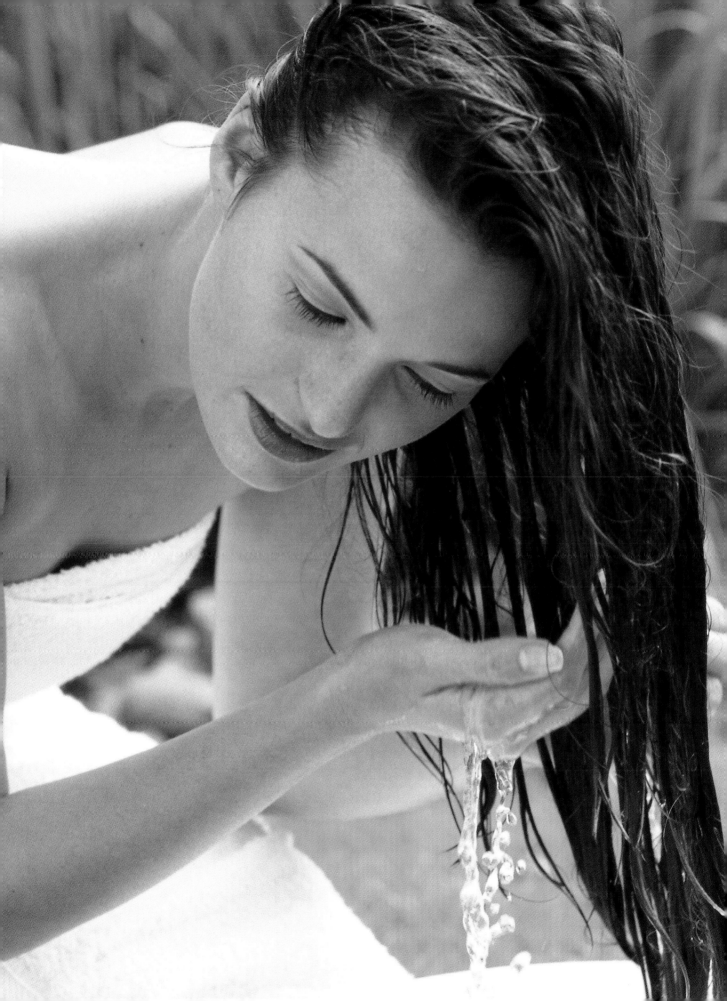

Back to basics

Shampoo is the most basic of haircare products, designed to clean your hair and scalp. (The word shampoo, interestingly, has its origin in the Hindi word *champi*, which means 'head massage with oil'.) Most shampoos are classified as detergents, with the exception of dry, powder shampoos that are less effective and tend to leave hair dull-looking. These can be useful, however, when you are not able to use normal shampoo because of your location or lack of time. Some shampoos contain soap, but most, these days, are soap-free and contain agents known as surfactants, otherwise known as surface-active agents, that lather well in all types of water. (Soap shampoo forms a scum with hard water.) Most modern shampoos also contain conditioning agents to make it easier to comb your hair after washing it.

A good shampoo should spread easily over the hair, rinse out, not irritate your skin or eyes and leave your hair manageable. The lather is not actually essential to clean your hair efficiently, but it does offer a guide to how much detergent you are using.

There is a wide range of shampoos for different hair types. If you wash your hair frequently or have

◀ *Shampoo is the most basic haircare product. A good one should spread easily over your hair, rinse out easily and leave your hair manageable.*

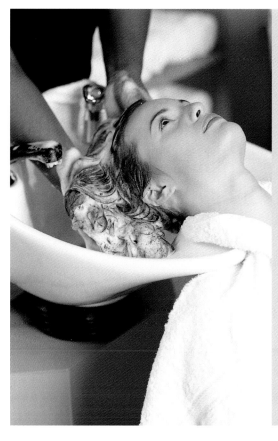

What's in shampoo?

■ Cleansing agents (surfactants). The two most common are ammonium lauryl sulphate and ammonium laureth sulphate, the milder of the two.

■ Conditioning agents.

■ Additives to control pH and thickness of the shampoo (if it is too runny, it would be messy to apply; if it is too thick, it would be hard to spread). Shampoos are usually slightly acidic, with a pH between 3.5 and 4.5.

■ Preservatives to prevent the shampoo from going off or ingredients from decomposing, which could lead to bacteria multiplying, and pose a health risk.

■ Colourants, perfumes and other ingredients to make the shampoo enjoyable to use.

■ Some shampoos such as antidandruff preparations contain zinc pyrithione.

a sensitive skin, choose a gentle formula. For colour-treated, permed or dry and brittle hair, a moisturizing shampoo may help. There are also special shampoos available for coloured hair but in truth they cannot really prevent colour fade, although they do moisturize the hair and help to maintain its condition. There is ongoing debate about the benefits of clarifying shampoos, which are used (normally about once a month) to remove so-called product build-up on

the hair. Some hair experts dismiss them, saying that a good regular shampoo should be able to remove all build-up of dirt and products on the hair anyway.

There are also many special formulations for greasy, dry and normal hair as well as shampoos for blonde hair that are designed to help it appear brighter.

Wash your hair as often as you need to – daily if necessary – but do not use too much shampoo, as it

won't make your hair cleaner! Brush your hair before you wash it – this loosens dead skin cells and any dirt sticking to your scalp.

Harsh sunlight, wind and other environmental hazards, as well as styling and chemical treatments, can damage the outer cuticle cells of your hair leaving it dull, dry and tangled. Unfortunately, conditioner cannot repair such damage but it can improve the appearance of the hair by coating the shaft, smoothing rough cuticle scales as a result, and making the hair easy to comb. Once the cuticle scales are flattened your hair also appears shinier. Whatever a manufacturer may claim, no conditioner can be absorbed into the hair shaft.

Always apply conditioner to freshly washed hair that has been patted dry with a towel. You need about a tablespoon of conditioner for short hair; double that for long hair. You can also massage conditioner into the scalp if the skin is dry and needs nourishment. Thereafter, comb it through the hair, concentrating on the ends. Rinse your hair very well after conditioning, as it can end up looking dull or even a little oily if you don't. After patting your hair dry detangle it gently with a comb.

Light conditioners are ideal for normal, healthy hair, and make it easy to detangle with a comb after washing. Intensive conditioners do the same job as regular ones, but are specially designed for dry, difficult to manage hair. Creamy, oil-based conditioners can improve the appearance and feel of dry hair. Volumizing conditioners can help fine hair to appear fuller. Very curly African hair needs to be particularly well-conditioned, as it tends to be dry and fragile. A gentle shampoo should be coupled with a rich conditioner.

Leave-in conditioners are less time-consuming than the types that have to be rinsed out and are designed to protect hair against heat damage and reduce static. To protect your hair from harsh sunlight, try a leave-in conditioner containing zinc oxide.

While nothing, except for a haircut, can cure split ends (the result of the outer, protective cuticle being stripped away or damaged) protein conditioners can smooth them temporarily, making them less obvious.

Types of conditioning treatments include: sprays, used before you style your hair to protect it against heat damage and to banish static electricity; and hot-oil treatments to deep condition dry and damaged hair. Regular hot-oil treatments are recommended for African hair.

Two-in-one shampoos – containing both cleansers and a high percentage of conditioners – were first introduced to the hair-cosmetics market in the 1980s, by pharmaceutical company Procter & Gamble. Their benefits, or lack thereof, were at first rather hotly debated, but these days about a fifth of all shampoos sold are two-in-one formulations that make use of silicones to carry out their dual task.

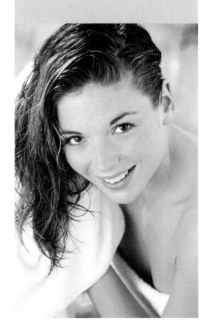

Did you know?

■ Dry hair stretches by a third to a half of its original length before breaking. Wetting a hair increases its elasticity, but also decreases its strength.

■ You should wash your hair as often as you need to. Daily washes will not cause sebaceous glands to produce more oil.

■ According to L'Oréal, 80 per cent of North Americans and 90 per cent of Japanese wash their hair twice a day, while the average frequency for washing hair in Europe is three times a week.

Tools of the trade

There is an array of styling products on the market. Here are some guidelines to help you choose.

CURL-DEFINING SPRAYS

As the name suggests, these are products for curly hair – they help to define your curls so that they do not go frizzy.

HAIR GEL

Gel comes as a transparent jelly or spray and can be used to mould damp or dry hair. It also gives lift to roots and structure to curls. The key is to use it sparingly: if you use too much you may end up with messy, sticky hair and have to wash and style it again.

Gel works better on coarse than on fine hair. It is good to control frizz and combat static electricity.

Mousse gives body and volume to hair – apply it from the roots to the ends. ▶

HAIRSPRAY

Hairsprays, quick-drying solutions containing polymers, are used to hold your hairstyle in place. They can also be used to reduce static electricity and give lift to your hair roots.

Look for the spray to suit your needs; options range from light to firm hold. Take care not to use too much or your hair could end up looking stiff and unnatural.

MOUSSE

Mousse is foam that gives body and volume to hair and is, therefore, particularly good to use on fine hair.

Choose a mousse to suit your purposes; some formulations offer firmer hold than others. Put the mousse on your hair from the roots to the ends before, or while you style your hair. It works especially well on curls and with diffuser drying or scrunching.

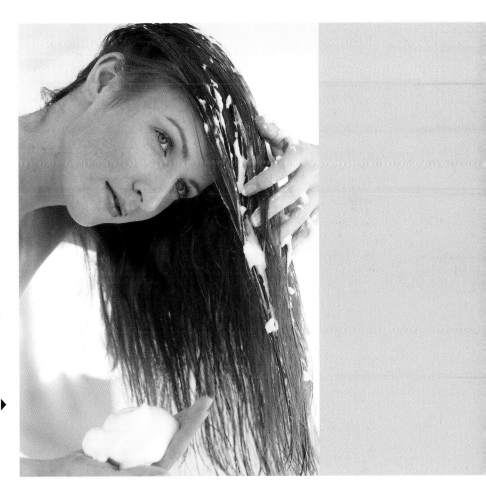

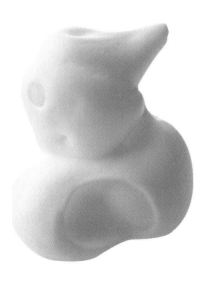

SERUMS, GLOSSES AND SHINE SPRAYS

Serums, glosses and shine sprays contain silicone or oils that form a microscopic film on the surface of the hair, boosting shine.

Use them on dry hair as the final step in your styling routine. They achieve the best results on sleek, straight hair. Some of the heavy serums can feel quite oily, so they should be used sparingly. Serums can help to fight frizz and make split ends less obvious.

STRAIGHTENING BALM

Straightening balms are used to protect your hair while using straightening irons or blow-drying frizzy hair straight.

STYLING LOTIONS

Styling lotions are designed to help your hair set into a particular shape. They are applied to wet hair, before you start styling. Some of them also protect hair against heat damage.

VOLUME ENHANCERS

Volume enhancers are specifically designed to add volume to limp, fine hair by coating the hair shafts.

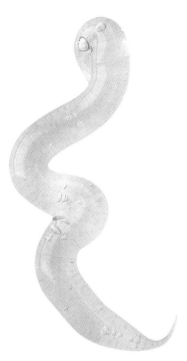

WAXES AND POMADES

These products are great on African, thick and dry hair. Skip them if you have fine hair. They also help to control curly, unruly strands and are useful in humid climates, where moisture in the atmosphere tends to make hair frizz despite your best efforts to control it.

Rather than fight your natural kinks and curls, use wax or pomade to sculpt them into something spectacular. Waxes and pomades must be used sparingly, as too much can make your hair look dull. They come in different strengths – gentler pomades generally provide a more natural look.

The right tackle

A regular grooming and beauty routine is unthinkable without all the right tools. Just pick your preference.

BRUSHES

If you are serious about styling your hair, invest in a number of hair-brushes with different purposes. Large paddle brushes are great for detangling long hair. For straight-forward brushing, flat brushes are the best, but you need a round brush for effective blow-drying. If you have short hair, it is easy to use a thin brush, while a brush with a larger diameter achieves the best results with long hair. If blow-drying is part of your grooming ritual, invest in a vent brush with a hollow centre. This allows hot air to flow through and assists with the process. The longer your hair, the larger the brush should be.

Also consider the bristles, which can be either natural (hog bristle) or synthetic (nylon, plastic or metal). Natural bristles are less damaging, but often too soft to brush through thick hair. Brushes with rubber balls on the tips of the bristles are kinder to your hair and scalp than those without. A hairbrush and curly hair are not compatible – use a wide-toothed comb instead. If you are losing your hair or have very fine and soft hair, stick to a soft natural-bristle brush.

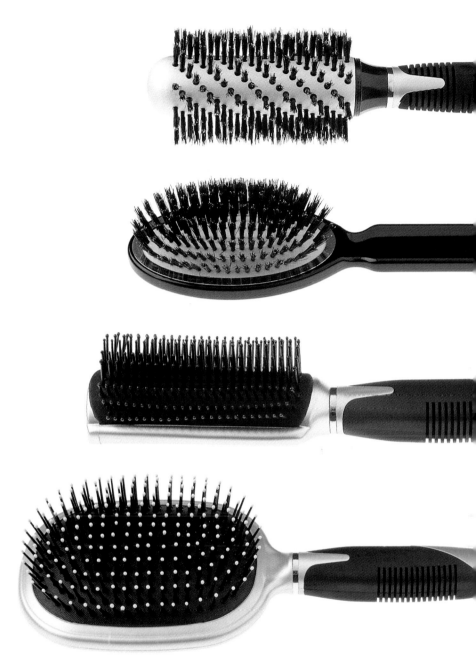

▲

There is a hairbrush for every purpose – from round brushes for blow-drying to paddle brushes for grooming.

COMBS

Grooming combs come in many shapes and sizes, with fine or wide teeth.

Long, widely spaced teeth are great for African, permed or very thick and curly hair, while regular wide-toothed combs are good to comb fragile wet hair or to detangle curly or permed hair. A tail-comb (with fine teeth and a long, thin tail) is used to make partings or to section off hair for blow-drying.

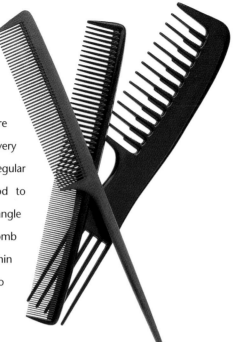

Use a tail-comb to create partings, a wide-toothed comb for curls and a regular comb to detangle knotted hair.

Do not use electrical hair appliances on chemically treated hair. The heat can damage the hair further and cause split ends.

Getting a head start

There is probably little truth to the claim that head massage aids hair growth but it does help blood circulation – and it is blood that brings nutrients to the hair-forming cells in the hair follicle. It can also help to relax your scalp and, in effect, release tension in your entire body.

Many salons provide scalp massages. If you want to try it at home: after you have applied conditioner, use your fingertips to gently rotate sections of your scalp, starting at the forehead and moving on to the sides, crown and finally the neck. Then place your fingertips on a section of the scalp and knead without moving your fingers. Do this for a short while and then move on to the next section, and so on.

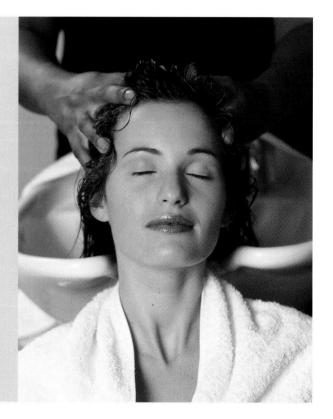

44

Hair extensions

Hair extensions are nothing new. In the late 1800s, fashionable upper-class women in Europe regularly used false hair to enhance their own. The hair came from young nuns whose heads were shorn upon entering convents, from prisoners and from poverty stricken young women who sold their hair for income. Modern-day extensions consist of real human hair or acrylic strands that get glued onto your own hair.

Professionally done extensions can add volume, length and colour to your own tresses, and change your image. They can easily be removed with solvent when they need replacing (after three months), or when you tire of them, but are not a long-term solution. Extensions attached by a qualified hairdresser should not damage your own hair or scalp and you can wash your hair as you normally would. If glued-on extensions seem too drastic, you can always experiment with temporary ones that clip onto your own hair. Just remember to hide the clips under your hair.

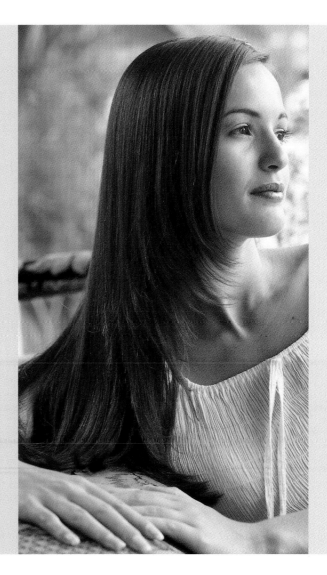

CRIMPERS AND STRAIGHTENERS

Like curls, crimping goes in and out of fashion. Crimping devices that consist of two ridged plates to produce ripples in the hair can be tough on hair, so limit their use and do not use them on damp, bleached or damaged hair.

Chances are, if you have naturally curly hair, you will yearn for rod-straight tresses. Blow-drying is the most common way of achieving this, but straightening irons – resembling crimpers with flat plates instead of ridged ones – have also become popular in recent years. To do their job well, straighteners need to be very hot, so make sure you protect your scalp (and your ears!) while using them. Even if fashion calls for poker-straight hair, try not to use straighteners every day. Crimpers and straighteners should always be used with heat-protective styling sprays.

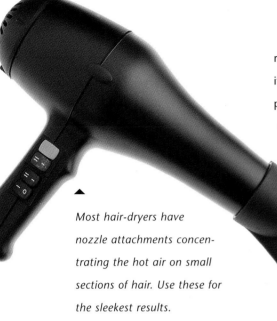

Most hair-dryers have nozzle attachments concentrating the hot air on small sections of hair. Use these for the sleekest results.

HAIR-DRYERS

It is worth investing in a quality hair-dryer if you blow-dry your hair regularly. A good blow-dryer has several heat settings: high heat for fast drying (but limit the use of this setting, as it is most harmful to your hair), medium heat to finish off your style and cool air to set it.

Hair-dryers come in different strengths, but 1200 watts should suit most people's requirements. Use a diffuser – which comes as a separate attachment – for curly or permed hair. The diffuser fits on the dryer's nozzle to gently spread the airflow so that your curls keep their shape.

To protect your hair, do not blow-dry it when it is sopping wet. Instead, remove the excess water by blotting it with a towel. Apply the styling product of your choice (preferably one offering some heat protection) and blow-dry your hair section by section. Most hair-dryers have a nozzle attachment that concentrates the hot air on a small section of hair – use this attachment for a straight and sleek result.

Always blow-dry down the hair shaft, so that the outer cuticle cells are pushed flat (which makes hair look healthy and shiny). Do not continue until your hair is bone dry; this is a sure way of damaging the hair shafts as removing too much moisture can lead to brittleness and breakage.

HOT BRUSHES AND HOT TONGS

Hot brushes and hot tongs should be used only on dry hair – both for safety's sake and to protect your hair.

A hot brush has bristles and, essentially, works like a standard brush combined with heat to help with styling. Take care when you wind your hair onto the hot brush, particularly if it is long, as it can easily get tangled.

A question of styling...

Hairstyling that does not involve chemical processes such as perming or highlighting is temporary, and sadly lasts only until the next shampoo. The reason is that, while your hair's keratin structure is permanently changed when you have it chemically treated, you can only alter it for a short period when you blow-dry your hair, or use hot curling or straightening irons.

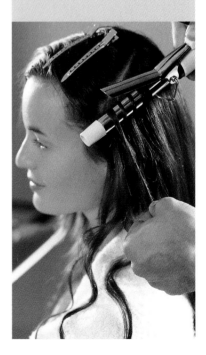

Hot tongs – which do not have bristles and are used primarily to create curls – come in different diameters. They can get very hot, so always make sure you protect your scalp when using them.

ROLLERS

If you often use conventional rollers choose smooth or foam-covered ones, which are less hazardous to your hair. The type with Velcro covering may be easy to use as they stay in your hair without clips, but they are almost inevitably difficult to remove, pulling out and breaking some of your hairs in the process. Thin curlers give tight curls, while thick ones create wavy hair.

Heated rollers – which come in sets and are heated on metal posts – work like conventional rollers and are good for giving volume while

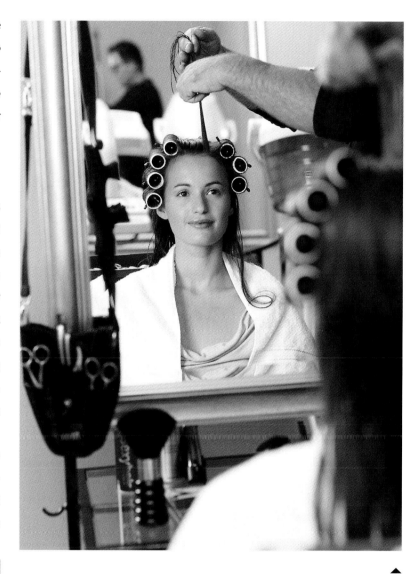

▲

Even if fashion calls for straight hair, do not use straighteners every day and always use heat-protective styling sprays.

creating curls. They work in a fraction of the time taken by conventional rollers. Choose the new types, which do not have potentially hair-damaging spikes. Use them on dry hair and remove them once they are cold, which can be in as little as 10 minutes.

Smooth or foam-covered rollers are less hazardous to your hair than Velcro-covered ones.

Protecting your locks

The multilayered structure of hair makes it strong and resilient, but your hair can only take so much before it will inevitably start to show signs of damage or weathering.

Obviously, chemicals used in solutions to straighten, perm or colour hair are some of the biggest culprits when it comes to hair damage. In addition, dermatologists worldwide have warned against the dangers of plaits that are made too tightly, particularly where fragile African hair is concerned – as these very often lead to scarring and hair loss. It is important to note that this is not only an adult problem: children may look very cute with tightly braided hair, but such styles may not be good for their future hair and scalp health.

The chemicals used to straighten, perm or colour hair are some of the biggest culprits when it comes to hair damage.

The age of individual hairs naturally plays a major role when it comes to health and shine; the longer your hair, the more years it has been exposed to all sorts of hazards and the more difficult it is to maintain, and to keep split ends at bay.

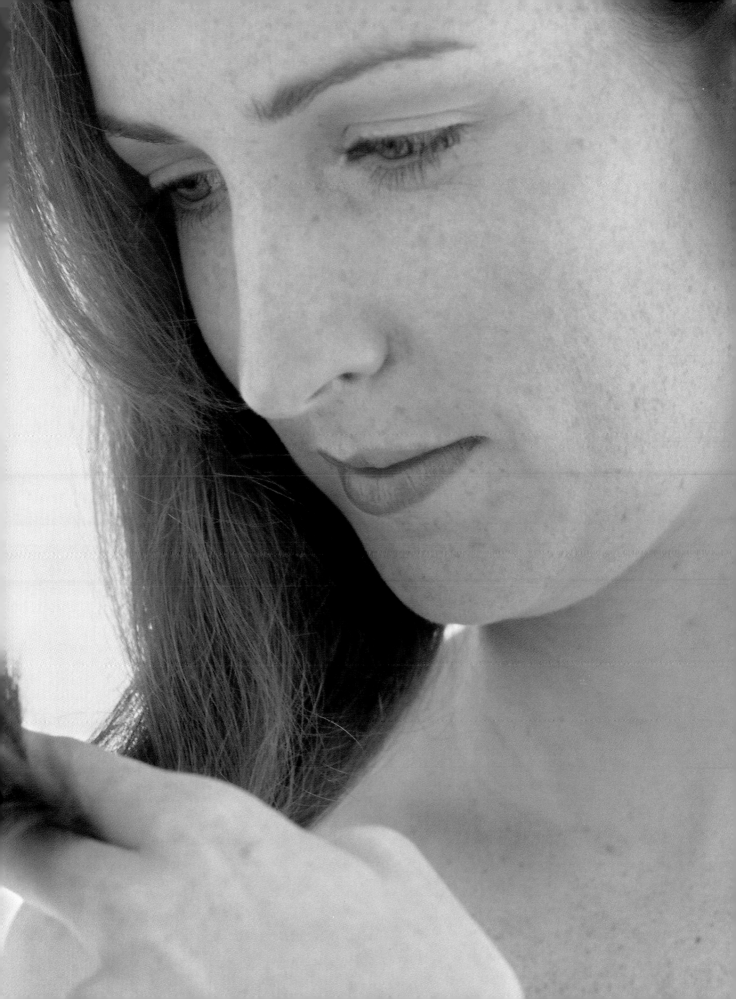

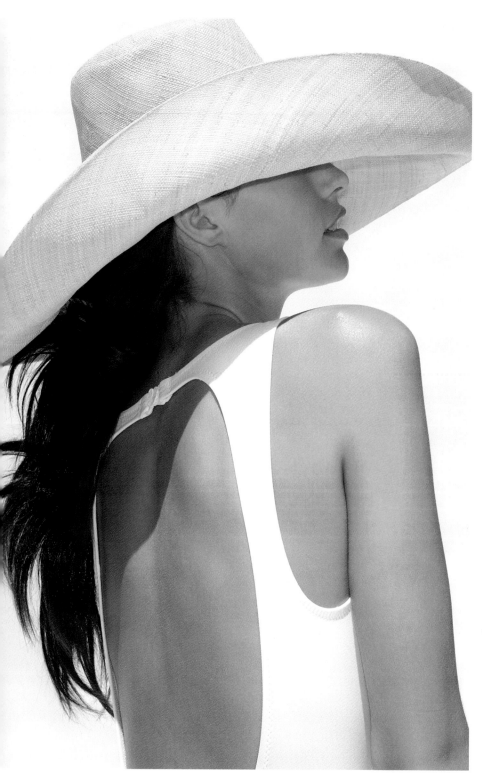

The great outdoors

Just as the weather and your lifestyle impact on your general health, these factors also affect your hair. The sun can bleach your hair, strip it of moisture and weaken its protein structure, while wind knots and tangles it, causing split ends and damaged cuticles.

Protect your locks by wearing a hat or bandanna when you are out on a hot, sunny day. When it is windy, tie up long hair to keep it from knotting.

Many hair products these days contain sun-protection ingredients. Unfortunately, many are not effective as their contact with the hair is too short to make a real difference, but if you can find a leave-in conditioner containing sunscreen, use it liberally on the beach or at the poolside.

◀ *Wear a wide-brimmed hat to protect your tresses against harsh sunlight, which can bleach your hair, weaken its protein structure and strip it of moisture.*

Alarmingly, blonde or highlighted hair tends to turn a shade of green after prolonged exposure to swimming-pool water, the result of a chemical reaction with the chlorine. Experienced hairdressers advise using tomato sauce as a solution for green hair. Just apply, wait a while and rinse off.

To prevent this from occurring, renowned trichologist Philip Kingsley's advice is to comb a water-resistant product through your hair before you go swimming. You can make your own by mixing together some high-factor sun protection oil and hair conditioner. This protects your tresses from the harmful effects of chlorine as well as salt water, and

Bad hairdressing methods are a common cause of hair loss and hair damage, particularly when it comes to fragile African hair.

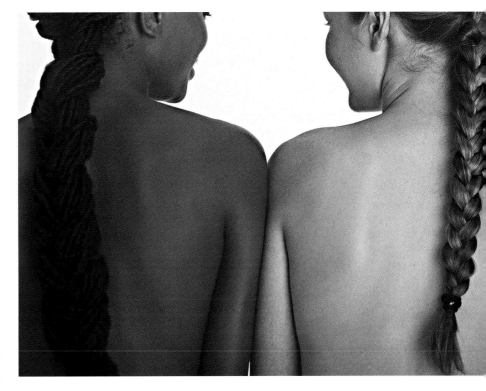

helps to maintain the moisture levels and condition of your hair. Also, remember to rinse your hair well with clean, clear water after swimming to get rid of chemical or sea-salt build up, or better still, wear a swimming cap.

Lastly, air conditioning not only dries the air, it also has a drying effect on your hair. Use a humidifier. Alternatively, a do-it-yourself option is to place a bowl of water near the air conditioner to replace the moisture that is taken out of the air.

▲

Tying up long hair in windy conditions protects it against knotting.

Styling sense and healthy hair

Bad hairdressing methods are a common cause of hair loss and damage, and devastating results are particularly widespread when it comes to fragile African hair. Tight braids, comprising your own hair or hair extensions, the misuse or overuse of chemical hair products, and constant pulling on the hair can all cause a condition known as traction hair loss or traction alopecia, prevalent among African and African-American women.

Traction hair loss often starts with the hair thinning at the front hairline, and then spreads. Balding can also occur in a band around the scalp, known as banded traction alopecia.

Chemicals used for straightening or 'relaxing' hair are potent and if not used properly – or overused – can burn the scalp. Serious burns can even destroy hair-follicle cells. Known as scarring traction alopecia, this condition in itself not only leads to hair loss, but also to inflammation and swelling of affected areas on the scalp.

Scarring traction alopecia is common and a much-discussed issue in dermatological circles. The consensus is that early diagnosis and a change in hairstyling habits are crucial to combating this problem.

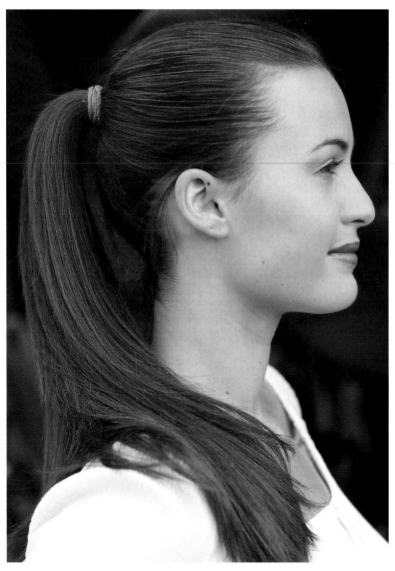

◀ *Tight ponytails can cause traction alopecia. Never pull your hair back so tightly that your scalp hurts.*

All this does not mean you should never consider braiding or relaxing your hair. If your hair is in good condition, a skilled hairdresser using good products can get excellent results.

Alarm bells should ring, however, if you notice hair damage or loss. In this case, reconsider your styling methods immediately. Remove tight braids or stop straightening your hair, and take preventive and restorative action (otherwise you may well be on the road to permanent hair damage, hair loss or scalp problems). Remember to condition your hair often to combat brittleness, brush relaxed hair with a natural-bristle brush, and never use unprotected and thin, elastic hair bands that can cut into your hair, damaging it and sometimes even intertwining with it. Thicker, fabric-covered bands are far better to gather your hair.

Sleeping in rollers, and repeatedly using heated rollers and electrical hot brushes, straightening devices and other appliances can also lead to hair damage and patchy hair loss. They are also known to lead to the phenomenon known as 'bubble hair'. This is caused by using the hair-dryer on too high a setting, or overusing other heated appliances. The heat causes the water inside the hair to boil, and results in the formation of little bubbles. The hair eventually breaks off at, or near, the bubble.

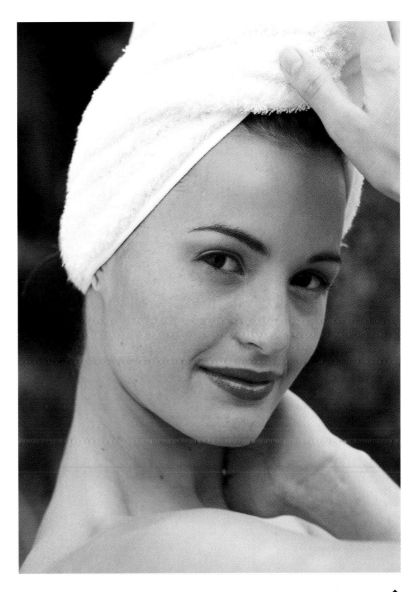

▲

When towel drying your hair, do not rub it vigorously. Blot it with a towel instead.

A question of chemicals

Let's face it, it is better not to perm your hair, but since perming also has its cosmetic benefits (such as giving volume to fine, thin hair and making hair more manageable), there will always be a need – and a case – for it, if it is done professionally. Modern products, while doing the same job as their predecessors, are gentler on your hair and less likely to damage it.

The strong and flexible keratin protein structure of hair makes it possible to style it in a variety of ways. Temporary styling – such as blow-drying and the use of electrical styling appliances – works on weak bonds between atoms in the long chains of amino acids that make up keratin. These weak bonds – mainly of hydrogen – can be temporarily broken by water or even humidity. As they break apart when hair gets wet, and form again during the drying process, these bonds give hair flexibility, because the bonds tend to form again in different places, changing its shape. For example, wet hair left to dry naturally ends up looking different from hair wound onto a brush and blow-dried.

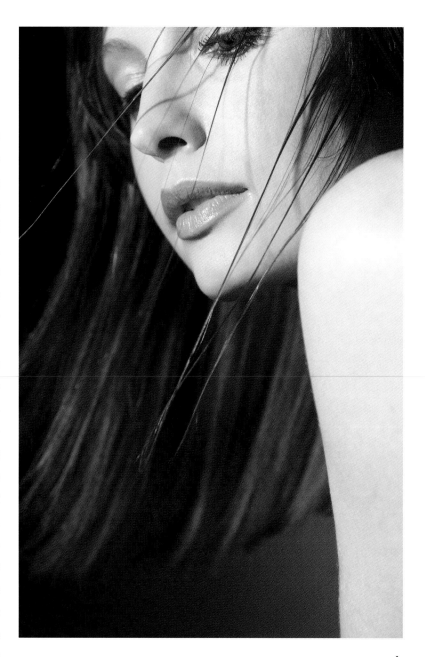

(This is why your hair looks a mess if it gets wet in the rain or if you don't control the drying process!) If you want to permanently alter the structure of your hair, however, you need to

New straightening methods, such as thermal restructuring, are much easier on the hair than traditional chemical straighteners.

tackle the strong bonds of hydrogen in your hair, which can only be broken through the use of chemical compounds. These bonds – which are, in fact, some of the strongest found in nature – are disulphide bonds (or disulphide linkages or bridges). By breaking them, you make straight hair curly (by means of a perm) and curly hair straight by means of chemical straightening.

PERMS

Perming works as follows: a hairdresser applies a slightly alkaline liquid – a curling fluid which contains reducing agents – to the hair to break down the strong disulphide bonds. The most commonly used reducing agent is ammonium thioglycollate. The hairdresser winds the hair around curlers to create the curls, which are then fixed with an acidic oxidizing solution, normally containing hydrogen peroxide (a neutralizing agent that fixes the chemical bonds in their new positions). The degree of curliness depends on the diameter of the curlers.

Perms are best done professionally so choose a reputable salon. A skilled stylist who applies the neutralizer at exactly the right point so that the perm is fixed with as little hair damage as possible can save you a lot of anguish!

One of the reasons care has to be taken during perming is that the scalp is vulnerable while, and after, the chemical solution is applied to the hair. Perming damage can also be minimized by using a quality product. (The scalp is even more vulnerable during straightening.)

To get the best out of a perm, make sure your hair is in the best possible health, and deep-condition it several times in the weeks preceding the perm. Do not use chemicals on your hair if you have a scalp condition or any sores on your head. Importantly, once it has been permed, do not wash, vigorously brush or blow-dry your hair for two days to make sure the keratin has properly hardened into its new shape. Use conditioner after every wash. If you want to get a home perm, follow the instructions carefully – it is important that every step is carried out as indicated. Remember, the temperature of the room can increase the speed at which the chemicals work, so be careful with them and do not keep them on your hair too long.

Do not perm and colour your hair on the same day as this will most certainly damage your hair. If you really need to perm and colour your hair, do the perm first, at least a week or two before the colour. A good salon should always do a patch test before perming or colouring your hair to assess whether there will be any serious hair damage, or allergic reactions to the dye..

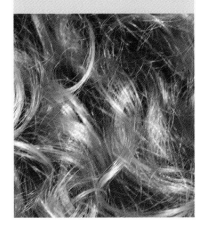

Among the perms available are body perms, using large curlers to produce soft curls and volume; root perms, designed to give volume only to the hair-root area; spiral perms, creating masses of spiral curls (best on long hair) and spot perms, targeting only certain areas, for example the crown or areas around the face.

A relatively new development is the semipermanent perm that gives volume to hair but does not last long. Modern products are gentler on the hair than those used a few decades ago, but do step up on deep-conditioning treatments, use a diffuser on your hair-dryer and never brush your permed hair – use a wide-toothed comb instead.

STRAIGHTENERS

The permanent straightening or 'relaxing' of curly hair works on the same principles as a perm and the reduction and oxidation process is similar but instead of winding hair on curlers, hairdressers comb it out straight from root to tip to uncurl it and then apply the neutralizer.

To straighten frizzy or kinky hair – such as African hair – alkaline products (like sodium or potassium hydroxide) are used. As they can harm the scalp,

they are suspended in thick creams. Sodium and potassium hydroxide definitely have a weakening effect on hair and make it far less elastic than untreated hair. There is also the danger that the traction of combing the hair can pull it out or break it off.

If you're having your hair straightened, go to an experienced professional. Also consider thermal restructuring, also known as Japanese hair straightening, thermal reconditioning or bio-ionic therapy (marketed as delivering negative ions to the hair).

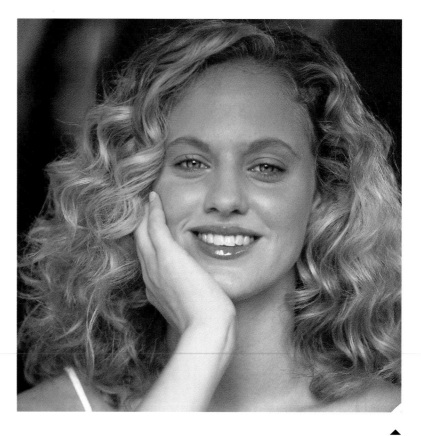

▲

This woman has had a successful body perm, which has given her lovely hair volume and has produced soft, loose curls.

To colour or not to colour?

Certain types of hair colouring, such as temporary tints, are not damaging to your hair, but bleaching and highlighting can adversely affect its condition. This is because chemical treatments alter the hair's cortex and affect its elasticity, which means that the hair stretches only to a limited extent and breaks easily when groomed.

Permanent colouring normally makes use of two solutions – one is the bleach to remove existing colour and the other is the new colouring agent. Bleach, commonly an ammonia or hydrogen peroxide solution, strips colour from your hair. When applied, it damages the hair's protein structure, giving it a characteristic brittle texture. It is thus recommended not to bleach or highlight your hair too often. Similarly, the more drastic your colour change the worse the brittleness will be.

Bleaching also makes hair more porous and vulnerable to other chemical

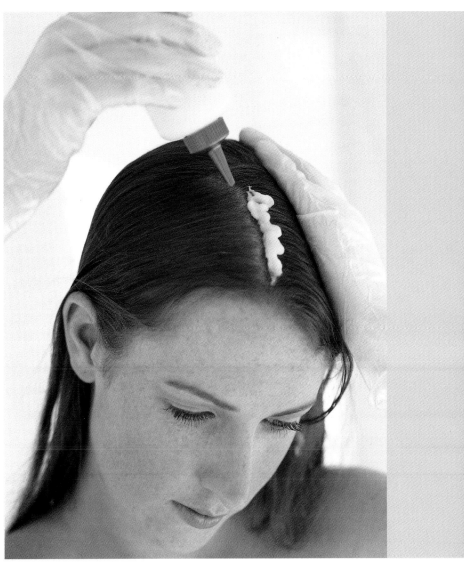

▲

A change in hair colour can really lift your spirits, but make sure you use a good product and follow the instructions carefully.

processes. This may cause irregular colouring as dry, porous hair absorbs colour too quickly.

Ensure your hair is in very good condition before you apply permanent colour to it, and thereafter, remember to condition it after every wash.

HIGHLIGHTS

Highlighting is a process during which small sections of hair are bleached. The old-fashioned way to do this was to pull strands of hair through a pierced cap. These days, sections of hair are normally wrapped in foil. Only a portion of the hair is bleached, so the process is less harmful than bleaching a whole head of hair, and it doesn't need to be done as often. However, repeated highlighting can still lead to damaged and dry hair.

Highlighting used to consist of two processes: the application of bleach, followed by rinsing, and the application of the required colour. Nowadays the two processes are combined using products containing both bleach and colour.

With permanent tints and highlighting, make sure you only have your roots touched up when necessary, so that the same hair does not get repeatedly blasted by drying chemicals.

On the upside, expertly done colouring can not only give you a fresh new look, it can also combat greasiness and make fine hair look thicker, as it swells the hair shaft.

Permanent solutions through the years

■ The first perms were done at the start of the 20th century, when chemicals, combined with high heat, produced 'permanent' curls. The early experiments led to scalp burns and hair breakage.

Fortunately for us, 'cold permanent waving', which did not require heat, was introduced in the 1940s. It is still the basic process used today.

■ Hair damage through styling is not a modern phenomenon. In the 1970s, L'Oréal, in collaboration with the Judiciary Identity Laboratories, studied 33-centuries-old hair taken from the mummy of the Egyptian pharaoh Ramses II.

They found that his hair – unsurprisingly – had been badly damaged. Although the passage of time was partly responsible, some of the damage was attributed without much doubt to his rudimentary combs.

■ Thick hair is easier to perm than thin hair. Perming solutions developed for Caucasian hair are diluted for use on Asian hair.

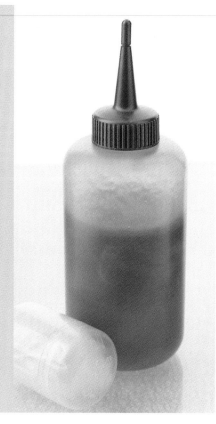

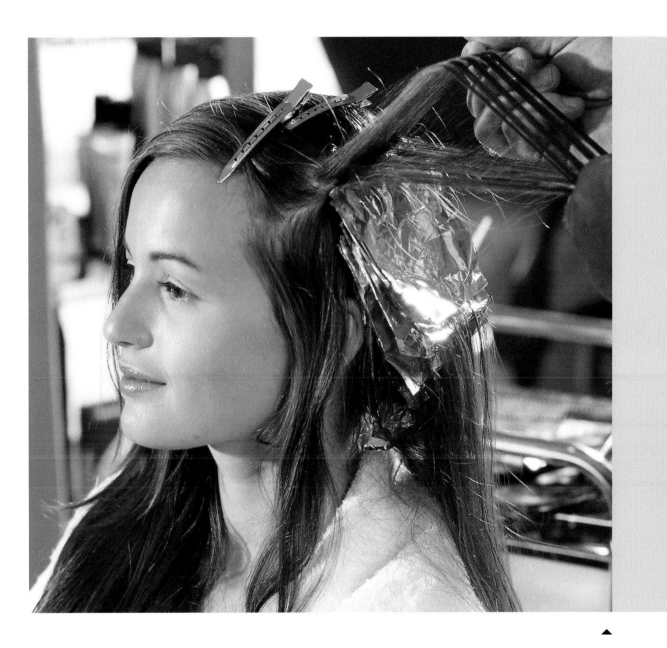

*During highlighting, small sections of
hair are wrapped in foil
and bleached.*

A natural alternative

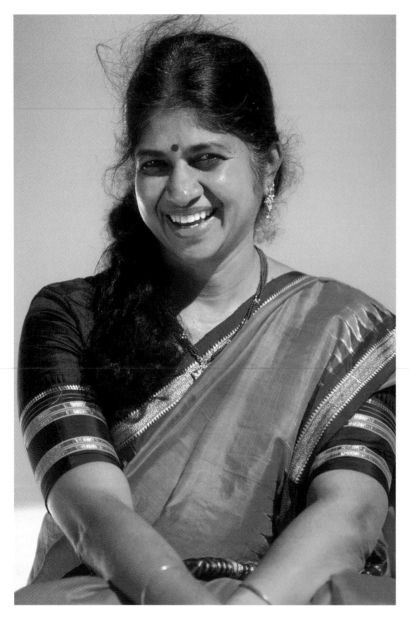

Henna, the most well-known natural hair dye, extracted from the Egyptian privet (*Lawsonia inermis*), is widely used in India and the Middle East. It comes as a powder that is mixed with water to form a paste, and works much like a semipermanent colour, staining the outside of the hair shaft.

While it does not have the damaging effects of chemical dyes, it can be difficult to predict the colour you will get. It is definitely best used on dark brown and black hair, to which it imparts a red glow. The longer you leave henna on your hair, the more intense the resulting colour will be.

Never be tempted to use henna on blonde, grey or highlighted hair – unless you don't mind a scary orange! Other natural dyes are chamomile and tea leaves.

Although henna is regarded as very safe, people who suffer from asthma and allergies should take care when using it.

▲

Henna, a natural hair dye regarded as very safe, is widely used in India and the Middle East.

Is it safe?

While some doctors advocate that you wait until the first trimester of your pregnancy has passed before you dye your hair, authorities such as the UK-based Oxford Hair Foundation conclude that dyeing your hair during pregnancy is safe.

Sceptics point out that – while there is no proof that chemicals in hair dyes are dangerous during pregnancy – there are also no reliable studies proving them to be safe. If you're worried, avoid dying your hair during the first trimester.

Highlighting hair is considered safer than colouring your whole head (particularly when using a dark colour). Vegetable-based products, such as henna, are also considered safer.

Concern about a possible link between dark hair-colouring products and cancer is nothing new. In fact, the hair dye industry has, in recent years, stopped using several ingredients that have been found to cause cancer in animals. There is, however, little concern that some of these dangerous compounds have now been replaced by chemicals with very similar structures.

Adding to the debate is a new scientific study conducted by Yale University researchers and published in the American Journal of Epidemiology at the beginning of 2004, which indicates that women who have been colouring their hair for some 24 years or more, starting before 1980, are a third more likely to develop non-Hodgkin lymphoma.

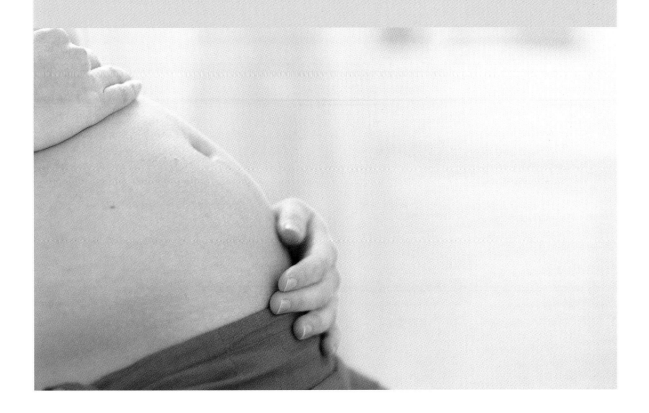

Getting your hair right

One of the most exciting things about hair is that you can change it so easily. Up to a point, you can play around creatively with what nature has given you; but not every style and colour is ideal.

The following guidelines should help you decide whether a certain style or shade would suit you but there are really no hard and fast rules. While your particular facial shape may call for a short cut, you may in fact detest short hair and feel more confident with long tresses. In that case, there is no point in chopping off your crowning glory. Your personality also plays an important role: that trendy cut and bright colour may theoretically suit you, but if you generally prefer not to draw too much attention to yourself, anything too wild may make your life a misery.

Up to a point, you can play around creatively with what nature has given you but not every style and colour suits everyone.

If you are planning a major change, talk it through with a hairstylist, who should be able to advise you on what will complement you and whether it will actually be possible to achieve a certain look with your hair type.

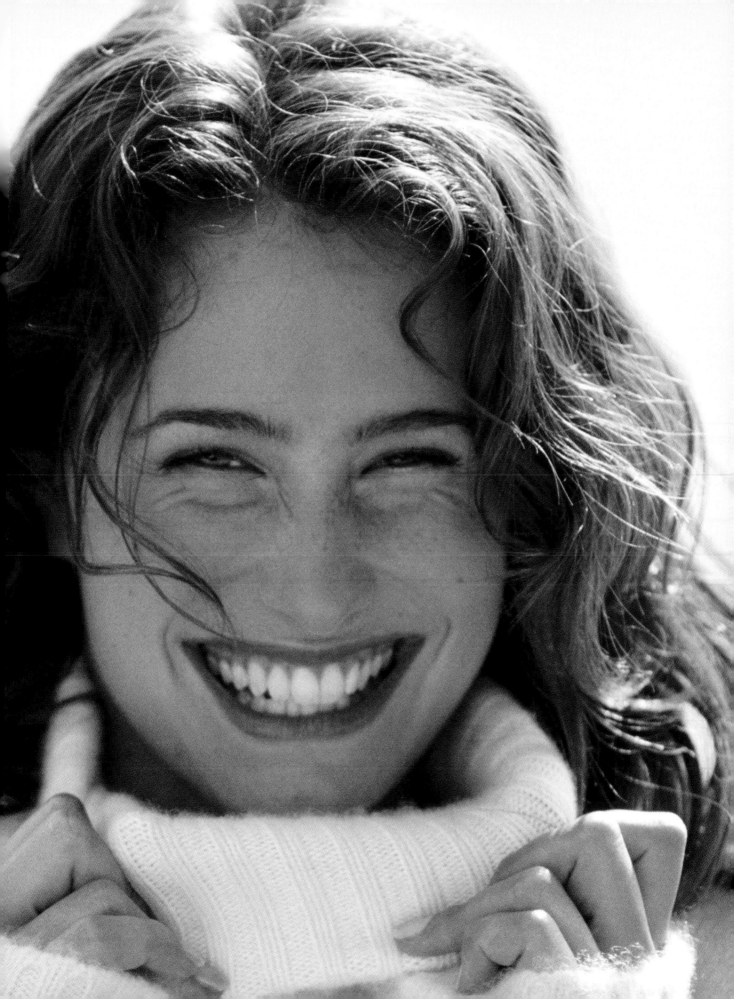

Your face the canvas

Hairstylists mainly distinguish between curved and angled faces. Curved or contoured shapes include oval, round, pear-shaped and heart-shaped faces. Angular face shapes include diamond-shaped, square, rectangular (long) and triangular faces.

If you are not sure what your facial shape is, tie back your hair, look straight into a mirror and trace the outline of your face on the mirror. Hopefully the shape will become clear to you. Remember, though, that how you see yourself is not exactly how other people see you – your side profiles and three-quarter profile are as important (prominent features being your nose and chin) as the full-frontal view.

The most desirable facial shape – from a hairstyle point of view – is the oval face. If you are lucky enough to have been born with an oval-shaped face, you are likely to be able to wear any hairstyle of your choice. In fact, stylists like to create the illusion of an oval face, for example, by 'broadening' and 'shortening' a rectangular (or long) face.

If you have a long face, the idea is to optically shorten it by wearing a fringe and/or layers. Preferably avoid long, straight hair, as this can accentuate the length of your face.

A heart-shaped face tends to be wide at the forehead, with a narrower jaw line. A hairstyle that narrows the forehead, but widens the

DIFFERENT FACE SHAPES

There are basic guidelines that can help you to choose the most flattering style for your facial shape, but do remember: side and three-quarter profile are also important.

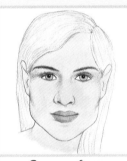
Square face

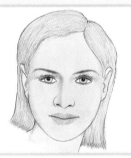
Oval face

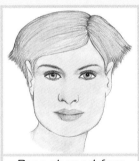
Pear-shaped face

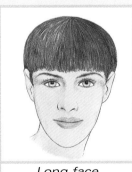
Long face

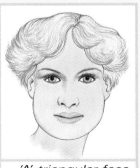
'A'-triangular face

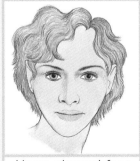
Heart-shaped face

This woman has an oval to slightly heart-shaped face to which her hairstyle gives perfect balance.

▶

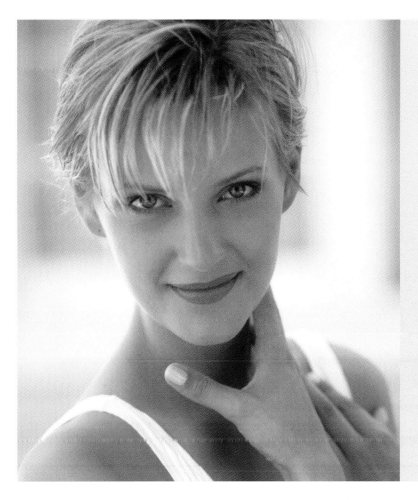

jaw line – with curls or waves, for example – should be a good choice. In this case, hair no longer than shoulder-length should be flattering. (The same goes for a diamond-shaped face.)

A pear-shaped face is just the opposite of the heart shape. In this case, you should attempt to widen your forehead and narrow your jaw line. Hair that is fuller around the forehead, with a narrowing effect at the jaw, should create good balance.

For both a round and square face, stylists recommend a style that will lengthen and narrow your face shape. This you can do by creating height with your hairstyle. A round, curly style will let your face seem even rounder – instead keep the sides short or long, sleek and close to the face. For a square face, try a side parting to draw the eye away from the square-ness of your face. Soft waves can create softness for a square face. Avoid severe hairstyles, such as a straight bob, which can make your look hard.

There are two types of triangular faces – the V-triangle and the A-triangle. The 'V' is widest at the forehead and thus needs less hair in that area and more around the chin (a round bob could work well), while the 'A' needs a style that is fuller at the forehead, for a widening effect. You may also have a combination of facial shapes, so use your common sense. A simple guideline to remem-

ber is that where your face is at its widest, avoid bulk or volume. (Keep your hair straight or tucked behind your ears, for example.) Where your face is narrow, use volume or layers to create width. Also, bear in mind that there should be a balance between the shape of your face and the rest of your body. (Masses of long hair are unlikely to suit someone who is short and petite.)

A question of colour

Just like no two faces are the same (except for those of identical twins), no-one else has exactly the same hair colour as you. Even black has subtle shade differences – determined by the type and amount of melanin in your hair. Changing your hair colour is a great way of reinventing yourself, but, again, there are some guidelines to bear in mind, the most important of which is your basic skin tone, which can be warm ('yellow') or cool ('blue').

If you are pale-skinned, a good way of determining whether your skin tone is warm or cool is to inspect the freckles on your arm. If they appear to have a charcoal colour, you are likely to have a cool skin tone. If they look honey-coloured or orange, your tone is warm. If you have dark Mediterranean skin or black skin, you are also likely to have dark eyes and dark hair, but you, too, can have a yellow (golden) or blue undertone in your skin.

Generally, you should go for warm hair colour if your skin tone is warm (with golden or reddish tones) while a cool colour should suit you if you have a cool skin tone (with a bluish undertone). Also remember that, while a certain shade of blonde, red or brown may not suit your complexion at all, another may do wonders for it.

Lastly, it is not only your skin colour that should act as a guide, your eye colour is also important. If you have dark eyes and skin, dark

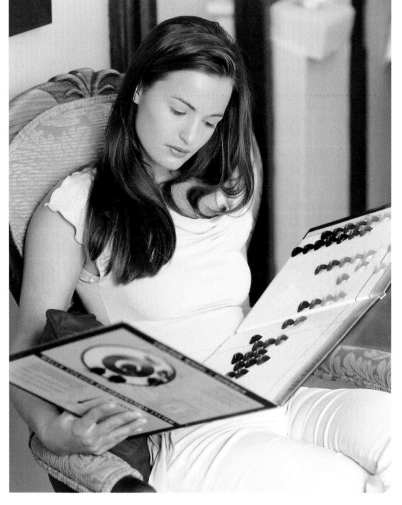

◀ *When it comes to hair colour, you have a wide choice, but do make sure you choose a tint that suits your natural colouring.*

Salon products vs. store purchases

This is a thorny issue. Many – if not most – salon owners swear that the expensive salon products on their shelves are far superior to their supermarket counterparts.

Is this really the case though, or should you save your money? Several dermatologists believe salon products are not necessarily superior in any way, apart from the more expensive and exclusive packaging. Many contain simple ingredients, such as salicylic acid, and products with a similar make-up can be bought less expensively elsewhere. Even when it comes to medicated shampoos, you are able to find products that are as effective as their salon counterparts on the supermarket shelf.

As stated earlier, the cleansing agent sodium laureth sulfate is gentler than sodium laurel sulfate, so a product containing the former may be a better choice. You will find plenty of supermarket products containing sodium laureth sulfate. Some manufacturers use natural ingredients or honey as a selling point. This may sound nice, but does not necessarily have anything to do with the effect of the product on your hair.

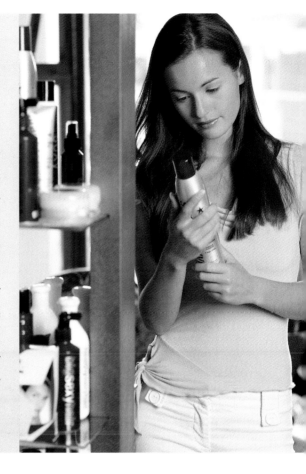

hair looks fabulous. Light eyes with dark skin? Then keep your options wide open, but light eyes combined with light skin generally calls for a lighter hair colour.

■ If you want to go red, but have a cool skin tone, burgundy, mahogany and similar shades will work for you. If your skin tone is warm, choose oranges, Titian or pure red.

■ If you want to go blonde, choose a gold or honey-blonde for a warm skin tone. Ash-blonde, Nordic blonde or beige are good options for a cool skin tone.

■ If you don't have a dark complexion or naturally dark hair, it is generally a bad idea to dye your hair pitch black, as it is likely to make you look older and paler. There are always exceptions, though. Typical pale Irish skin is very well complemented by very dark hair, for example. Not everyone can go very fair either – particularly if you have very pale eyes you may end up looking rather washed out. (However, good make-up may solve this problem.)

■ Solid colours that are very blonde, or dark, are generally not flattering unless you have very clear skin. They can also look unnatural, particularly if you are using it to disguise grey.

■ Highlights are a great option if you don't want to dye your whole head, but are not suitable for everyone.

Highlights look best if you have fair or medium brown hair, but steer clear if your hair is dark brown, black, or grey. (Lowlights – dark streaks, as opposed to light ones – work well with grey, particularly for men).

■ If you want to cover grey hair, don't choose a dye too similar to your natural hair colour. As you grow older, lighter colours may do more for your complexion. Temporary colour won't cover grey successfully; demi-permanent or permanent dye will.

Of course, the more radical the change, the more time-consuming it is likely to be to keep up your new colour, so consider your lifestyle and willingness to spend a fair amount of time at the hairdresser. (As an indication, if you choose a permanent colour that is far from your natural one, you may need to have your roots tinted every four to six weeks.) Also bear in mind the harmful effects the chemicals can have on your hair (therefore, only the roots that have not been in contact with dye before should be touched up).

Water-based temporary colours coat only the outside of your hair and are easily washed away. They contain no chemicals and do not harm the hair shafts. Temporary colours carry relatively fewer risks of allergic reaction than permanent colours do.

Semipermanent colours penetrate the outer cuticle scales of the hair and cover the inner cortex, but also wash away after six to 12 shampoos. You can only go darker or redder, as this type of dye cannot lighten hair (it does not contain hydrogen peroxide or ammonia).

Demipermanent colour lasts longer than semipermanent colour (up to 26 washes). It does not contain ammonia, so you cannot lighten your hair using demi-colour. It does contain a small amount of peroxide,

If you are a natural blonde, add a few golden highlights.

If you find your red hair dull, get some copper streaks.

To brighten up your black hair, consider a few highlights.

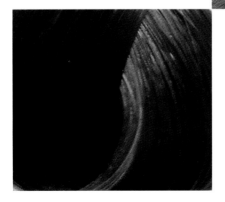

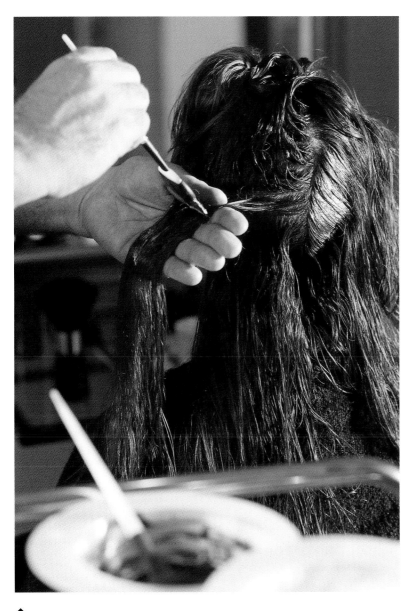

▲

Modern permanent colouring methods tend to be gentler on the hair than the older two-step process.

however, which opens up the cuticle scales so that the colour can penetrate the cortex to a certain extent. Demipermanent colour is very good to cover grey and, as it washes away, regrowth is not nearly as obvious as with permanent colour.

Permanent colour enters the hair's inner cortex, and a chemical reaction – brought about by ammonia and peroxide – results in a permanent change to the colour (until it grows out). The benefit of permanent colour is that it can make hair darker or lighter. It does not fade like semi-permanent colour.

Modern permanent colouring methods tend to be gentler on the hair than the older two-step process, during which hair was first stripped of all its melanin, and then dyed to a new colour using another chemical process. These days, a less concentrated bleach solution (containing about 20 per cent hydrogen peroxide) is used, in conjunction with a dye and cleansing agent, to achieve the new colour in one single step.

Getting rid of unwanted hair

Hair removal for cosmetic reasons is nothing new – the ancient Egyptians are believed to have used sugar and beeswax to remove superfluous body hair. The threading method of removing excess facial hair – which is still used today, particularly in the Arabian Gulf and India – is believed to be many centuries old. Archaeologists have also found instruments like sharpened rocks, suggesting that men shaved their beards many thousands of years ago.

In Elizabethan times it was considered extremely desirable for fashionable women to have high foreheads – this resulted in women plucking their front hair-lines to make their foreheads appear higher.

The threading method of removing excess hair - used particularly in the Arabian Gulf and India - is believed to be centuries old.

As your choice of hairstyle gives some indication of your personality; so too, your decision on whether or not to remove body hair makes a personal statement. And this does not only apply to women as an increasing number of spas and beauty clinics now cater for men. In particular, waxes and laser hair-removal treatments have become a unisex pursuit.

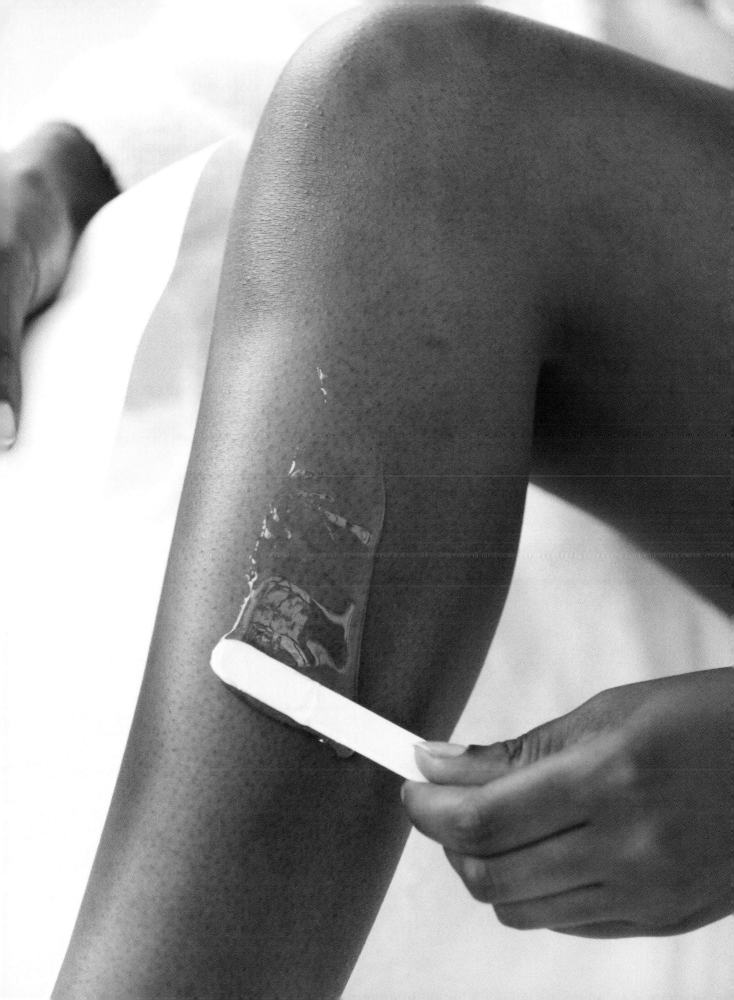

A guide to hair removal

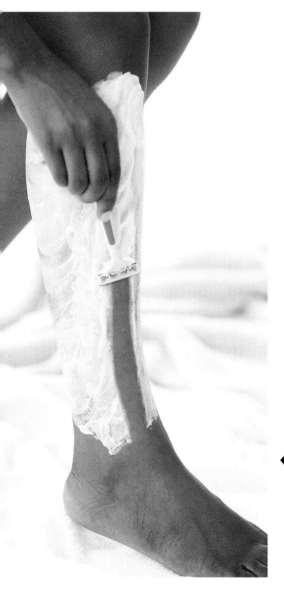

Hair can be removed temporarily through depilation (the removal of the part of the hair that is visible, for example by shaving or using depilatory creams) or epilation (removing the entire hair by plucking or waxing).

SHAVING

This is the most common and straightforward way of hair removal; particularly useful in getting rid of unwanted hair on legs or under the arms. Make sure you use a sharp blade and sufficient lather. Shaving can irritate the skin or lead to ingrown hairs on sensitive areas, such as the bikini line for women.

Contrary to popular myth, shaving does not make hair grow out darker or thicker and it does not stimulate hair growth. The hairs may feel prickly while they are growing out, but they are unchanged in every way once they are fully grown.

◀ *Use a sharp blade and sufficient lather when you shave your legs, as shaving can irritate the skin or lead to ingrown hairs.*

DEPILATORY CREAMS AND LOTIONS

These contain chemicals that easily dissolve the protein that makes up unwanted hairs. They work well for some people, but are not recommended if you have a very sensitive skin or are prone to skin pigmentation, as they can cause inflammation. If it is possible, limit the use of depilatory creams to your legs. Keep them far away from your face as even a mild chemical burn could cause hyper-pigmentation. (You could end up with a hairless but unsightly, pigmented moustache area, for example.) It is a very good idea to first test a patch of skin for possible irritation.

EPILATORS

Because rotary epilators pull hair out this process of depilation is very painful. Aside from the benefit that no chemicals are used, there are no advantages to using epilators. They are known to be ineffective in pulling out fine and short hairs, because the tweezers cannot grasp them, and those hairs that are seized tend to be broken.

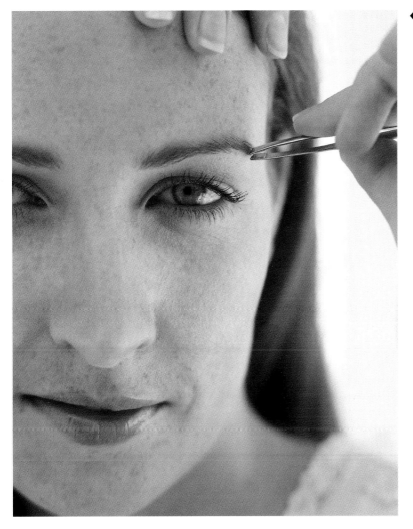

PLUCKING

Plucking (tweezing) is an effective way of pulling out individual stray hairs on the eyebrow area, and can be painful. (Never tweeze the hairs on the upper lip or chin, or those on a pigmented mole.) Always use a good quality pair of tweezers; an inferior one could break off hairs or tweeze your skin along with the hair. A benefit of this method is that, if tweezing is done correctly, it does not damage the skin and, like threading gets rid of stray hairs for two to four weeks.

Rubbing some ice over the area that you plan to pluck before you start may help to slightly numb the site, making it less painful.

THREADING

This is a very quick and effective, traditionally Indian and Middle Eastern, way of getting rid of rows of unwanted hair, but it is catching on in the West too. The therapist uses a piece of taut twisted thread to pull out the hair. It is no more painful than tweezing and is faster.

WAXING

Waxing – during which strips of hair are plucked out by their roots – is one of the most popular ways of salon hair removal (it can be done at home, too, but is better left to the professionals). It is known to be painful but effective, and many women – and men – keep going back for more! However, waxing can inflame sensitive skin and should not be used if you are prone to broken capillaries.

There are two types of waxes: 'hot' and 'cold' (although cold wax is also slightly hot to the touch when applied). Hot wax is a thick substance, generally used on sensitive areas, such as the face, bikini line and under the arms, while cold wax is much thinner and runnier, like syrup, and is usually used on body areas where the skin is less sensitive, such as the legs and arms. Ingredients include beeswax and paraffin.

As waxing plucks out the hair, regrowth is slower than with shaving. Side effects may include allergic contact dermatitis due to the colophony (a substance used in wax obtained from the sap of pine trees). Do not wax when you are on the drug Roaccutane (used to treat acne), as the waxing does not only remove the hair, but also a layer of skin. When you choose a beauty salon, make sure that the therapists are qualified and that hygienic practices are followed (some salons still recycle their hot wax after use, although this practice has been strictly outlawed).

ELECTROLYSIS

Electrolysis is a process during which the hair follicle is targeted by an electrical current from a very thin needle, causing localized damage to the dermal papilla. The hair is then simply removed with a pair of tweezers.

Electrolysis can be a very good tool to get rid of unwanted hair. However, make sure you choose a qualified and skilled practitioner, as the procedure can produce little white scars if not done properly. Also, it is a time-consuming process during which individual hairs are targeted and is only useful for small areas. (Since the arrival of laser hair removal, electrolysis has shifted into the background somewhat.) However, unlike lasers, electrolysis is effective for both dark and fair hair.

Take care to stay out of the sun – or use a very good sunscreen – for about

If you are considering laser hair removal :

■   See a dermatologist for an initial consultation to make sure you don't have an underlying medical condition.

■   Avoid fly-by-night clinics, or clinics not attached to certified medical facilities. It is best to be referred by a dermatologist.

■   Preferably have the treatment during winter, when your skin is paler than in summer.

■   For a month before laser treatment, stay out of the sun, use a high-factor sunscreen, and do not use self-tan lotions or sunbeds.

■   As laser treatment targets anagen hair (hair in their active growth phase), you should not wax, bleach or tweeze for six weeks before a treatment, and do not use any hair-removal creams either.

two days after having electrolysis, and keep perfume and chemicals away from the treated area. While having the treatment, you feel a tingling sensation in your hair follicle. The discomfort is more acute in sensitive areas. You repeat the treatments every six to 10 weeks.

It is safe to have hair removed from most parts of your body using electrolysis, as long as the skin is undamaged. Exceptions are the hairs inside your nose and ears, and those on pigmented moles.

LASER HAIR REMOVAL

The most revolutionary method of successful modern hair removal is, without a doubt, laser hair removal, and this technology is continually being fine-tuned and improved.

During the treatment, a laser, consisting of one wavelength and a pulse width of monochromatic light, targets the melanin in the hair (the darker the hair, the better). The aim is for the laser to destroy the hair follicle without harming surrounding tissue or causing hypopigmentation of the skin (areas of lighter pigmentation).

Laser hair removal is sometimes marketed as being permanent – although this is not the case, even though it can remove some hairs permanently in instances where the hair follicles are completely destroyed. (This is also the case with electrolysis). Unfortunately, not all hair follicles are targeted accurately enough to achieve permanent removal of all the hair. So, at most, you can expect hair reduction. You will also need multiple treatments over several months – how many, depends on the part of your body that you are having treated, and this

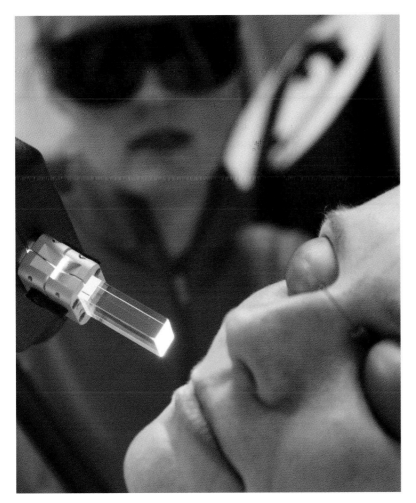

◀ *This woman is having laser treatment to remove unwanted hair from her face. Both she and the laser operator are wearing goggles to protect their eyes.*

also varies from person to person. The good news, however, is that laser treatment does delay hair growth, and scientific studies have shown that this may lead to temporary hair loss for about three months.

Because the laser targets the melanin, the treatment works best for people with dark hair (containing lots of melanin) and fair skin (containing little melanin), but as the technology improves, good results are also being achieved on darker skin (however, if you have very dark or black skin, laser treatment is definitely not for you). As you have to have pigment in your hair for laser hair removal to work, you are also not a candidate if you have blonde or grey hair.

One of the major benefits of laser treatment is that when it is done professionally, it is a safe procedure and can treat large parts of the body in a short period of time (as opposed to electrolysis where each hair is targeted individually). There are a number of excellent lasers for laser hair removal. The one best suited to you depends on your skin type and the part of the body that is to be treated. These days, dermatologists seem to prefer lasers with a slightly longer wavelength, such as the normal mode alexandrite laser, the pulsed diode laser and the YAG laser.

You have to wear eye protection during the treatment to prevent any possible damage to your retinas. Depending on your pain threshold, there is minimal pain. (Generally, you do not need anaesthesia, but for larger or more sensitive body areas, a topical anaesthetic, applied as a cream, should do the trick.) If you have dark skin, you may have some temporary hypopigmentation (lighter areas of pigmentation) following the treatment.

There is a risk of scarring if the laser practitioner uses too powerful a laser during the treatment – another reason to choose the best clinic you can find. Opting for a less reputable establishment offering inexpensive treatments may not save you money in the long run.

STICK TO THE TRIED AND TESTED

The treatments mentioned are established and medically approved methods of hair removal. However, if you do an Internet search – or scan the classified advertisements in certain publications – you may come across a number of other hair-removal methods, some not approved by medical bodies or scientifically tested.

Stick to the tried-and-tested techniques, and do not waste your money – or compromise your health – on bogus treatments. Some of these include electric tweezers (using electrified tweezers to apply an electric current to the hair), dietary supplements and 'hair growth inhibitors'.

Non-laser light hair removal

Non-laser light sources (also known as Intense Pulsed Light Source) produce a multiwavelength light and have been scientifically shown to effectively remove hair. (The technology has been marketed as EpiLight.) A specific wavelength can be chosen to suit your hair colour and skin type. Studies have shown about 60 per cent hair removal 12 weeks after a single treatment, but long-term studies are continuing.

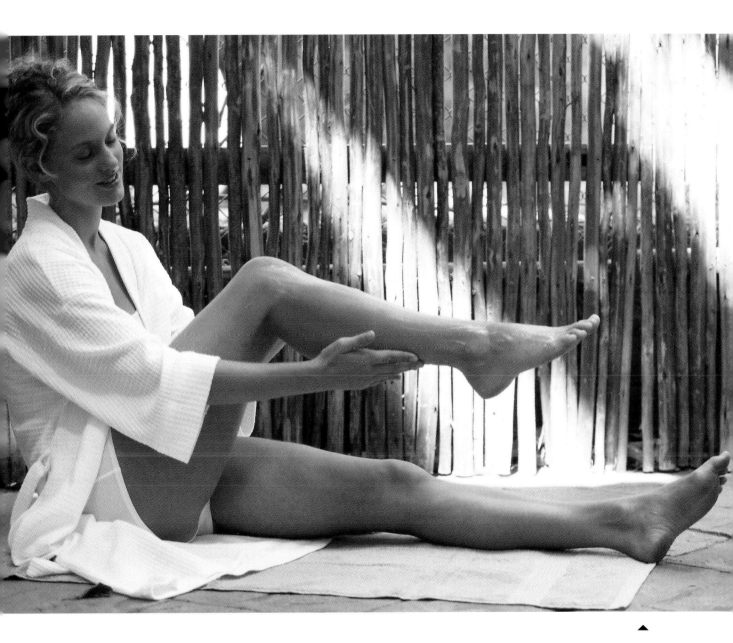

Silky-smooth, hair-free legs can be achieved in a number of ways – from shaving and waxing to using depilatory creams and lotions.

A male perspective

Human beings, according to the UK-based Oxford Hair Foundation, have more hair on their heads than any other species of primate, but researchers continue to debate its function and the reasons for men losing their hair in the case of genetic male-pattern baldness. The question is whether the hair on your head and face really serves a purpose in temperature regulation and sun protection (the counter-argument here is that humans have not kept the hair on their noses, which are particularly vulnerable to sun damage), or whether, in fact, it has more to do with sexual signals and attracting a mate.

Whatever the reason, men these days have a myriad options when it comes to styling, colouring and combating greying. Even when it comes to balding, you have safe avenues that could take years off your age and boost your self-confidence. Fortunately, a neat style is no longer limited to short back and sides – partly thanks to style icons like British footballer David Beckham modern men have been freed to literally let their hair down.

Men these days have a myriad options when it comes to styling, colouring and combating greying.

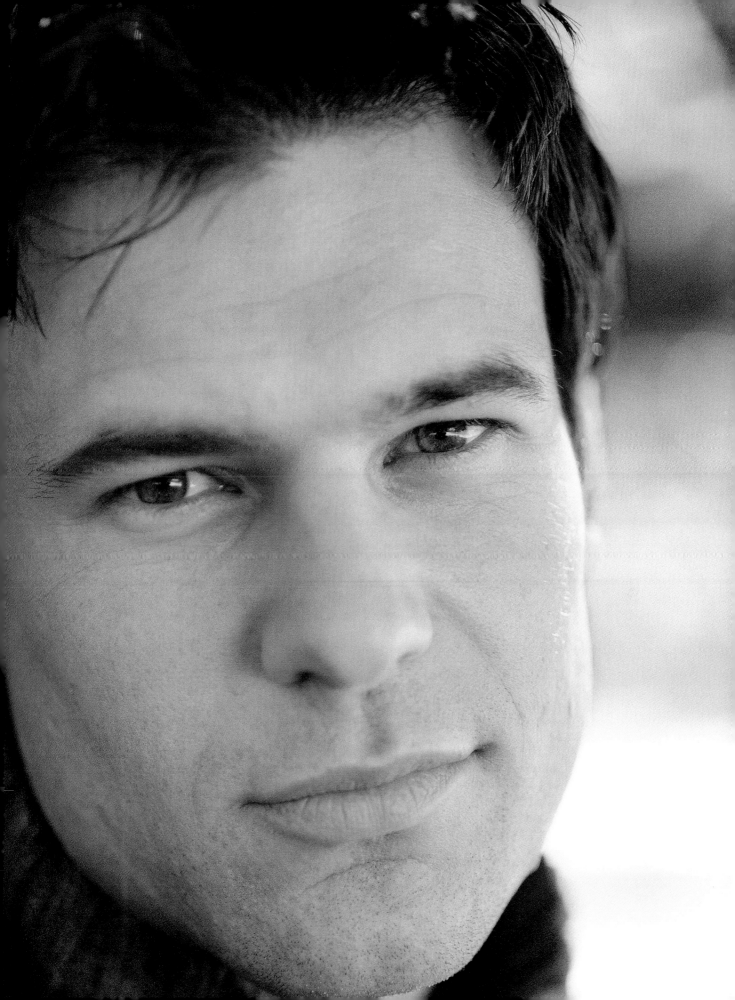

The best style for you

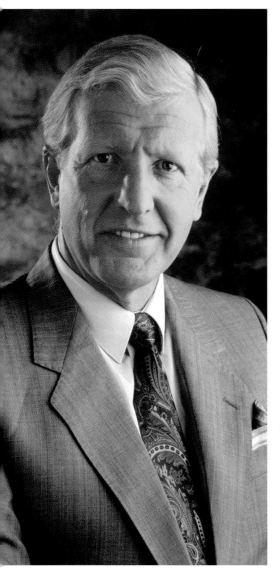

It is not only women who should consider their facial shapes when choosing a hairstyle – the same goes for men. However, where women have to make do with the hair on their heads, men can use beards or goatees, or even a moustache, to make the most of their features, or to conceal features considered less flattering. Just remember that a beard or moustache does not suit everyone, and that facial hair can be ageing. Your side and three-quarter profiles, as well as features such as a prominent chin, nose or ears, play a role when choosing a hairstyle. Longer hair at the sides can conceal ears that are large or stick out, while a big nose could be balanced by hair that is a little longer at the back.

As with women, an oval face is the ideal. If you have this facial shape, you are spoilt for choice. If you have a square face, most hairstyles will suit you – just keep your hair relatively short around the ears, so that the square look is maintained. If you have a long (rectangular or oblong) face, choose a style with a shortening effect. A fringe or layers could work wonders. A round face looks thinner when offset by a well-styled beard. Slightly longer hair could have a lengthening effect.

Hair that is a little longer at the back could work well to balance out a V-triangular face with a pointy chin. (Alternatively, a goatee could camouflage the chin.) If you have an A-triangular face, try a fringe or layers to create some bulk around your forehead.

You can have the best cut in the world, but not be able to maintain it if you are unsure of what products to use: a hair serum is best for a sleek style, for example, while a wax is good to control curly or frizzy hair.

◀ *Your hairstyle should suit your facial shape and hair type, but it is equally important to consider your personality, lifestyle and profession. This businessman's hairstyle helps to give him a professional and distinguished look.*

Style sense

There is no need to despair if you find your hair thinning or greying. Apart from the fact that these changes are completely natural, there are a number of ways that you can make the best of what you have.

IF YOUR HAIR IS THINNING:

If you are balding, the golden rule is to keep your hair short and neat – stylists advise that any hairstyle requiring you to comb long strands of hair over balding areas is a strict no-no. Have your hair cut by an experienced and professional hairdresser.

Not everyone can carry off the shaved-head look. Unless you are nearly bald, extremely handsome or a sporty type of man, you should probably steer clear of this. A good tip is that colouring thinning hair just one shade darker tends to make it seem fuller. Products that take the sheen off your scalp are a variation on this theme – they are based on the premise that your hair seems thicker if less of your scalp is visible. Some gels and sprays may make your hair seem thicker and fuller. A beard could give you a whole new look.

However, being bald or balding can be stylish these days – Hollywood superstars like Jack Nicholson and sport legends such as Andre Agassi are leading the way. Flaunt your pate by donning stylish eyewear, dressing well or sporting a trendy bandanna.

Male-pattern baldness starts with a receding hairline at the temples. Eventually only the hair at the sides and back may remain.

IF YOUR HAIR IS GREYING:

Greying hair is a natural part of growing older. Like balding, it is genetically determined. Caucasian hair tends to grey quickest – by the age of 50, 50 per cent of Caucasians find that half the hair on their heads is grey. Greying starts near the temples, the result of a gradual decline in melanin production.

Fortunately, most men look distinguished with a little grey in their hair. However, a good way of camouflaging your grey is by getting lowlights (darker streaks, the opposite of highlights). The result is often more natural than if you tint your whole head, and you need to have it done less often. This is because regrowth is less obvious, and blends in with the rest of the hair. If you know from the outset that you want to disguise your grey, do not wait until you are noticeably grey before doing something about it.

Although mainly aimed at women, there are a few home-colouring ranges for men. Remember, temporary colour doesn't cover grey; demipermanent and permanent colour does. (Permanent colouring is best done at a salon.)

Male hair-loss myths

■ The degree of baldness corresponds with the density of hair on the body.

■ There is no basis to believe that any link exists between male baldness and libido.

■ Male-pattern alopecia is caused by poor blood circulation. (Many bogus products marketed as combating hair loss are based on ingredients that would supposedly improve blood circulation and thereby stimulate hair growth or regrowth. Save your money.)

■ While it is true that starving or extremely malnourished people do tend to lose some hair, natural hair loss experienced by a healthy person on a reasonably good diet cannot be linked to diet. Hair-loss products containing amino acids, vitamins and zinc will therefore not stop your hair from falling out.

■ Hair loss cannot be caused by clogged pores, frequent hair washing or tight hats and helmets.

■ Laser treatment cannot cure baldness and does not result in regrowth. When lasers are used in conjunction with approved drugs some regrowth may occur – but most dermatologists tell you that this is thanks to the drugs and not the laser (practitioners at centres that promote the use of lasers to remedy hair loss may disagree).

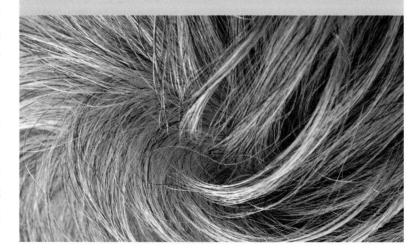

82

LOSING YOUR HAIR?

There are numerous possible reasons for hair loss (*see* Chapter 3), but by far the most common cause of thinning hair in men is male-pattern baldness (androgenetic alopecia). This starts with a receding hairline at the temples, followed by hair loss on the front of the head. In time, the bald patch enlarges, and eventually only hair at the sides and back of the head may remain. Eventually this hair, too, may fall out.

If your hair is thinning, bear in mind that this is such a common phenomenon that it is highly unlikely to bother anyone but yourself. Natural hair loss – even when premature – is not a medical problem and is entirely due to genetics. However, if you are one of many men who are willing to try almost anything to restore your locks to their former glory, the good news is that there are two drugs that may work wonders – minoxidil and finasteride – but only as long as you are having active treatment. A hair transplant may also be an option. Be under no illusion though – the vast majority of hair-loss remedies, including the much-touted laser therapy, are completely useless.

In case you have wondered, hanging upside down to improve blood flow to your head, rubbing your scalp with hot chillis and consuming vast amounts of vitamin and mineral supplements will not help.

Caucasians appear to be more prone to hair loss than Africans or Asians. It is estimated that up to 96 per cent of Caucasian men lose hair to some degree. According to research published in the Annual New York Academic Science, 30 per cent of them have androgenetic

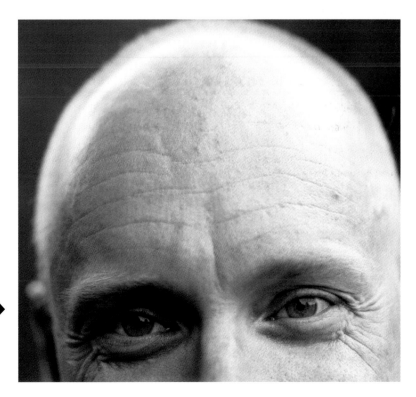

Some men lose all their hair within five years, but mostly it takes between 15 and 20 years. ▶

alopecia by the age of 30, and 50 per cent have it by the age of 50.

Male hair loss can start anytime after puberty, and some men bald much faster than others (again, this is genetically determined). Some lose all their hair within five years, but mostly it takes between 15 and 20 years.

How does it happen? Balding is partly the result of changes in the growth cycle of hair. The number of hairs in the active growth phase (anagen) starts decreasing, while more hair goes into the resting (telogen) phase. Also, long, dark, terminal hairs start to be replaced by short, unpigmented, vellus hairs. At the same time, 'miniaturization' of the hair follicles (reduction in follicle size) takes place. These events lead to increased shedding of hair and finer hair with less pigment being produced.

Male androgenetic alopecia is a progressive condition. You cannot stop it, although the two approved drugs minoxidil and finasteride may temporarily stop the process and result in some regrowth. Interestingly, not only humans tend to lose their hair. Orang-utans and chimpanzees reportedly also show some signs of balding after sexual maturity.

HAIR TRANSPLANTS

Hair loss as a result of male-pattern baldness is linked to the effect of the androgen dihydrotestosterone otherwise known as DHT, on susceptible hair follicles in men (and on those of a very small percentage of women) who are genetically predisposed to it.

Testosterone is changed to DHT by increased levels of a hormone known as 5(alpha)-reductase. (This interaction causes miniaturization.) The typical pattern of this type of hair loss clearly shows susceptible follicles to be concentrated at the top and front of the head, while the ones on the sides and back appear to be more resistant. Surprisingly, when hair from a part of the head that is not balding is transplanted to an area that is balding, the transplanted hair remains resistant to androgenetic alopecia. It is this characteristic that makes hair-transplant surgery possible.

The first hair transplants were carried out about 40 years ago. Up until the late 1980s, these transplants resulted in a look that became known as the 'corn-row' effect, whereby implanted hair was transplanted in neat rows using the now out of favour punch-biopsy method. The result was unnatural and accounts for a lot of the bad press that implants have received. Since then, techniques have improved

Top transplant tips

■ When choosing a hair-transplant clinic, thoroughly check the practitioners' credentials. Only consider the treatment if it is to be carried out by a skilled surgeon after an extensive consultation.

■ Ask to meet patients who have had the treatment and see results before you make up your mind.

■ Do not choose a clinic just because it offers less expensive treatments than others – you may pay dearly for your choice.

■ After the transplant, do not exercise for 10 days and avoid other activities that lead to sweating. Do not wash your hair for three days, to protect the implanted grafts.

vastly, and better results are obtained today. If done by a skilled surgeon, the modern way of implanting hair, by means of grafts, eliminates the 'corn-row' effect and leads to a natural-looking hairline.

How does it work? At the start of the process, a thin strip of skin with hair is taken from the area behind your ear. This donor skin contains follicles with hair that is not genetically programmed to be shed. The strip of skin is then dissected into tiny micrografts (containing one to three hairs) or minigrafts (three to five hairs). This is known as donor harvesting.

The donor area behind the ear is immediately stitched closed and covered by your existing hair. The harvested grafts are then painstakingly implanted into the skin in the bald area of the scalp or area where the hair is thinning.

The transplanted hairs or hair units are planted into the skin less than 1mm (0.03in) apart. Depending on your degree of baldness, the process may be repeated a few times to achieve the required hair density. The transplant is usually done under local anaesthestic and is not painful. It is a lengthy process, however, that can take up to six hours, as several thousand grafts may need to be implanted.

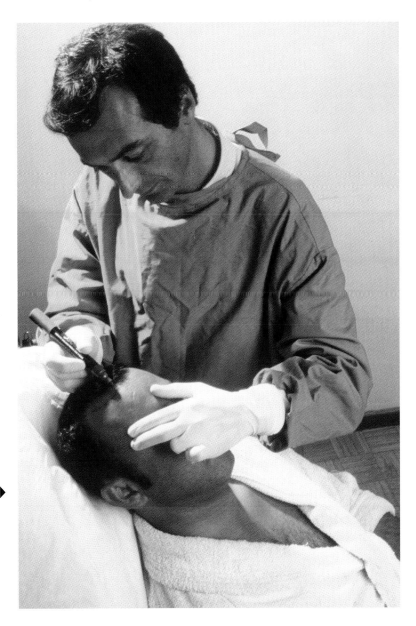

A hair transplant, usually done under local anaesthesia, is a lengthy process that can take several hours, as thousands of grafts may need to be implanted.

A hair-transplant surgeon painstakingly implants hair grafts into a patient's scalp.

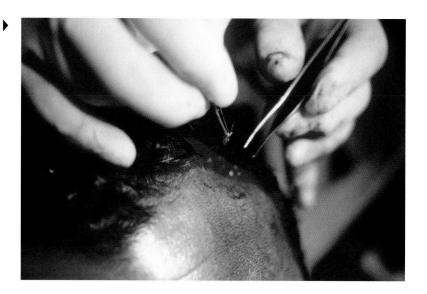

The healing process takes about 10 days, during which there is some redness and scabs form where the hairs have been implanted. Once the graft sites have healed, there should be no visible scars. Do not be alarmed when the hairs in the grafts fall out within 10 days to two weeks after the transplant – this is normal. In the following eight to 20 weeks, the implanted follicles recuperate and generate new hair, which starts growing normally, with hair cells actively dividing.

Bear in mind that your expectations should be realistic. During a hair transplant, no more hair is created, but the existing hair is simply spread around. So, the coverage depends on how many healthy hair follicles you still have. If you are totally bald, you are unlikely to be a candidate for a transplant. If you have little remaining hair, a transplant is not

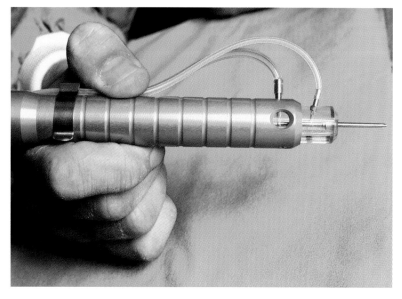

◀ During a hair transplant, this device is used to implant the hair grafts.

going to provide you with a luxurious full head of hair but – if your hair is thinning or you have a small bald patch – the transformation could be quite spectacular. The key is to have enough remaining hair so that it can be transplanted to bald areas of the scalp.

Only consider a hair transplant if your hair loss is natural or the result of other non-reversible causes such as traction alopecia or burns. If the loss is reversible and caused by factors such as thyroid disease, high fever, medication or infection, the answer is not a transplant: you need to have the cause established and treated. You don't have to wait until you reach a certain age to have a hair transplant. If you address the issue early, your balding will be less visible.

When considering a hair transplant, ▶
it is important to be realistic, as you
are not creating more hair, but
simply spreading the hair you still
have over a greater surface area.

The non-surgical option

Wigs and toupees have had bad press in the past, but modern hair systems – as they are known these days – should not be scorned. Made with human hair or quality synthetic strands, a good system can achieve a natural look. Fibres are usually implanted into a polymer material that looks like skin. (The older method involved the hair being tied into mesh bases.) The latest hair systems can be custom-made to match the client's natural hair colour and texture. The downside is that wigs and hairpieces are not permanent. Good ones are expensive, need a fair amount of maintenance and also need to be to be replaced regularly.

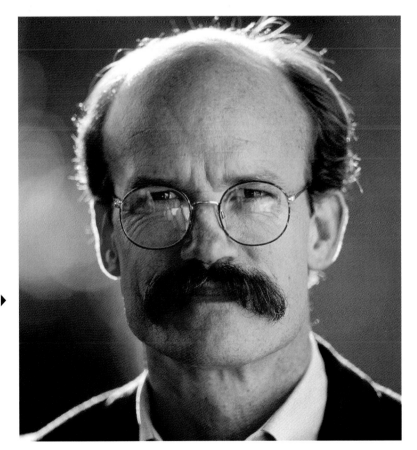

STYLE SENSE

Glossary

Alopecia: Hair loss.

Amino acids: Basic components of proteins.

Anagen: The growing phase of hair with constant cell production.

Androgens: Male hormones.

Catagen: The transitional phase of the hair-growth cycle, when the follicle stops producing hair.

Club hair: Hair in the resting stage which is ready to fall out.

Cortex: The central part of the hair which is packed with keratin.

Cuticle: The outer layer of cells protecting the cortex of the hair.

Dermal papilla: The part of the hair follicle where growth takes place.

Dihydrotestosterone: A derivative of the hormone testosterone.

Eumelanin: The dark pigment predominating in dark hair.

Hair bulb: The part of the hair cylinder surrounding the dermal papilla.

Hair shaft: The visible part of the hair.

Highlights: The lightening of fine sections of hair with bleach.

Follicle: A depression in the skin containing the dermal papilla where a new hair originates.

Keratin: The protein that makes up the consistency of hair.

Keratinocytes: The cells that form the keratin that makes up the consistency of hair.

Lanugo hair: The hair on an unborn baby.

Medulla: A central hollow core in some hairs.

Melanin: Hair pigment.

Oestrogen: Female hormone.

Phaeomelanin: The light pigment predominating in blonde and red hair.

Sebum: An oily substance produced by the sebaceous glands in the skin.

Surfactants: 'Surface-active agents' found in shampoos.

Telogen: The shedding phase of the hair-growth cycle.

Telogen effluvium: General hair loss from the scalp.

Terminal hair: Long, thick hairs that grow on the head and parts of the body.

Testosterone: Male hormone.

Traction alopecia: Hair loss as a result of strong traction (pulling) caused, for example, by braiding or ponytails.

Trichocytes: Cells in the hair follicle that divide to form hair.

Trichologist: An expert in trichology, the branch of medicine that deals with the scientific study of the hair and scalp (and their diseases).

Trichotillomania: A compulsion to pull out one's own hair.

Vellus hair: Short, unpigmented hairs.

Useful Addresses

CONTACTS

UNITED KINGDOM

- Oxford Hair Foundation

- Department of Dermatology,

Churchill Hospital, Old Road, Headington,

Oxford, OXS 7LJ, United Kingdom

- Website: www.oxfordhairfoundation.org

- L'Oréal (UK) Ltd

255 Hammersmith Road,

London W6 8AZ

- Tel: +44 20 8762 4000

- Website: www.loreal.com

UNITED STATES

- American Hair Loss Council

- 125 Seventh Street, Suite 625,

Pittsburgh, PA, 15222,

United States

- Tel: +1 412 765 3666

- Fax +1 412 765 3669

- National Alopecia Areata Foundation

- PO Box 150760, San Rafael,

CA 94915-076, United States

- Tel: +1 415 472 3780

- Fax: +1 415 472 5343

- Email: info@naaf.org

- Website: www.alopeciaareata.com

ONLINE CONTACTS

CANADA
- The Canadian Hair Research Council
- www.hairinfo.org/en/learning/disorders.html

EUROPE
- European Hair Research Society
- www.ehrs.org

INTERNATIONAL
- Keratin.com hair information source
- www.keratin.com

- Wella
- www.wella.com

UNITED KINGDOM
- Philip Kingsley
- www.philipkingsley.co.uk

UNITED STATES
- North American Hair Research Society
- www.nahrs.org

- Proctor & Gamble
- www.pg.com/science/haircare

GENERAL WEBSITES

- www.thehairstyler.com

- http://hairdos.net

- www.hairboutique.com

- www.worldofhair.com

References

The following books and journals were consulted as sources of reference:

Alora, M., Arndt, K., Dover, J., and Geronemus, R., *Illustrated Cutaneous & Aesthetic Laser Surgery*, Second edition. Appleton & Lange, 1999.

Dawber, R., and Dawber, R.P, *Diseases of the Hair and Scalp*, Third edition. Blackwell Science, 1997.

Gray, J., and Dawber, R., *A Pocketbook of Hair and Scalp Disorders*, Blackwell Science Ltd, 1999.

Grey, J., *World of Hair: A Scientific Companion*, Palgrave Macmillan, 2001.

Jose, A., *Love Your Hair*, Thorsons, 2002.

Kingsley, P., *Hair – An Owner's Handbook*, Aurum Press Limited, 1995.

Openshaw, F., *Hairdressing Science*, Longman Scientific and Technical, 1986.

Reader's Digest, *Foods that Harm Foods that Heal: An A-Z guide to Safe and Healthy Eating*, Reader's Digest, 1997.

Rudiger, M., and von Samson, R., *388 Great Hairstyles*, Sterling Publishing Co., Inc., 1998.

Schwan-Jonczyk, A., *Hair Structure*, Wella AG, 1999.

Stoppard, M., *Woman's Body, A Manual for Life*, Dorling Kindersley, 1994.

Wadeson, J., *Hairstyles. Braiding & Haircare*, Lorenz Books, 1994.

Wingate, P., and Everett, F., *Hair & Makeup*, Usborne Publishing, 1999.

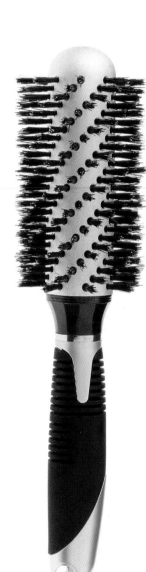

Photographic credits

All photographs by Micky Hoyle for New Holland Image Library (NHIL) with the exception of the following photographers and/or their agencies. Copyright rests with these individuals and/or their agencies.

(***Key to locations:** t = top; b = bottom.)

2–3	Digital Source		Warren Heath	65	Photo Access
4–5	Digital Source	33	Science Photo Library/	71	Ian Reeves/Shine Group
6	Photo Access		Susumu Nishinaga	72	Ian Reeves/Shine Group
9	Photo Access	34	Photo Access	75	Science Photo Library/
12	Digital Source	35	Photo Access		Michael Donne
13	Digital Source	40	Photo Access	77	Ian Reeves/Shine Group
15	Photo Access	50	Patrick Toselli	79	Photo Access
17	Photo Access	51	Photo Access	80	Photo Access
27	Photo Access	54	Patrick Toselli	82	Photo Access
28	Science Photo Library/	55	Digital source	85	Science Photo Library/
	Sue Baker	56	Ian Reeves/Shine Group		Mauro Fermariello
30	Science Photo Library/	60	Photo Access	86 t	Science Photo Library/
	Michelle Del Guercio	61	New Holland Image		Michelle Del Guercio/
31	Science Photo Library/		Library(NHIL)/	b	Science Photo Library/
	Lauren Shear		Ryno Reyneke		Mauro Fermariello
32	New Holland Image	63	Snapstock/Werner	87	Photo Access
	Library (NHIL)/		Bokelberg		

Acknowledgements

The publishers gratefully acknowledge the assistance of Marius Edgar of **FRONT COVER HAIR DESIGN** for giving us permission to use his beautiful facilities for the photo shoot as well as Karmen Lombard for the loan of her brushes and styling accessories.

Index

A

A-triangular face **64**, 65

African hair 16, **17**

air conditioning 51

alopecia 24 *see also* hair loss

alopecia areata 25, 26

alopecia areata totalis 26

alopecia areata universalis 26

ammonia 57

ammonium thioglycollate 55

androgenetic alopecia 24

androgens 26 *see also* male
hormones

Asian hair 16, **17**

autoimmune disease 25

B

baldness 22, 24, 52, 78, 84

banded traction alopecia 52

basal layer **10**

biotin 33

black hair colour 67

bleach 57, 58

blonde hair colour 67

blow-drying 43, 45

brushes 43

bubble hair 53

C

cancer 61

Caucasian hair 16, **17**

central medulla 10

characteristics of hair 18

chemicals 54—56

chemotherapy 27

childbirth 26

chronic illnesses 26

coarse hair 19

cold wax 74

colour 12, 57—59, 66, 67,
68, **69**

combination hair 21

combs 44

conditioners 40

contact dermatitis 29

corneal layer **10**

corn-row effect 84, 85

cortex 10, 18

   functions 11

cortisone injections 26

crimpers 45

curl-defining sprays 41

cuticle functions 11

cuticle **10**

D

dandruff 28, **29**

demipermanent colour 68, 82

dermal papilla 10

dermatophytes 28

diet 32—35

dihydrotestosterone 31, 84

disease 26

disulphide bonds 55

donor harvesting 85

dry hair 20

E

eczema 29

electrolysis 74

epilators 72

erector pili **10**, 12

eumelanin 12

F

facial shapes **64**, 80

female hormones 26 *see also*
   oestrogens

female-pattern hair loss 24

fever 27

finasteride 31, 83, 84

fine hair 19

flat brushes 43

furfuracea 28

G

glosses 42

grafts 86

grey hair 68

greying 19, 34, 82

growth cycle, anagen phase 11

   catagen phase 11

   telogen phase 11

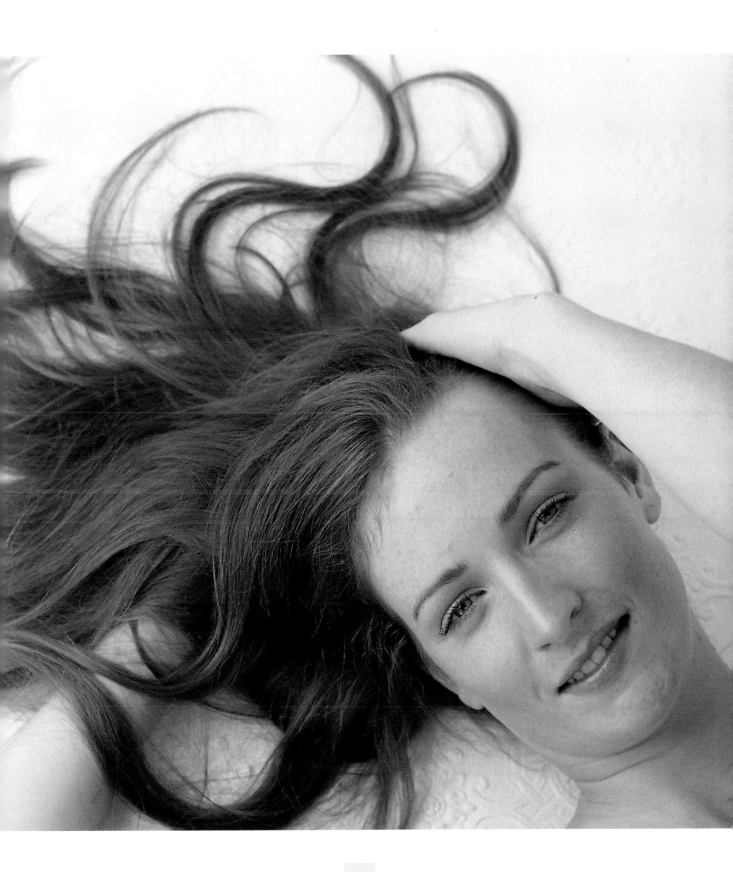